MW01232143

The Source® for TBI
Children & Adolescents

Paul C. Lebby, Ph.D.
Shana J. Asbell, Ph.D.

Content Area	Ages
■ Traumatic Brain Injury	■ 0-18
	Grades
	■ PreK through High School

Evidence-Based Practice
■ See Page 2 for evidence-based practice statements.

LinguiSystems

LinguiSystems, Inc.
3100 4th Avenue
East Moline, IL 61244
800-776-4332

FAX: 800-577-4555
E-mail: service@linguisystems.com
Web: linguisystems.com

Printed in the U.S.A.

ISBN 978-0-7606-0746-6

■ *The Source for TBI – Children & Adolescents* promises to be very useful for professionals working with brain-injured children and adolescents, including primary physicians, nurses, therapists, school teachers, and social workers. It also promises to be very helpful for family and friends struggling to understand TBI-related disability. This text fills a gap in available information about traumatic brain injury because it is concise without being oversimplified. It is well-organized and readable, with very helpful examples from the clinical setting. The material is soundly-based on current science and understanding of neurophysiology and pathology. The figures and up-to-date MRI images of children with TBI assist in illustrating the relationship between brain structures and functional limitations.

This work provides a clear discussion of cognitive impairments particular to children with traumatic brain injury, enriched by real-life examples. The discussions relating to the assessment and intervention of children with TBI highlight the authors' expertise in this area, and will be extremely helpful to therapists and school personnel who want to develop appropriate therapeutic and educational settings for children with TBI, whose needs are often not met in a classroom designed for children with developmental disabilities. The *LANSE-A* and *LANSE-C* are particularly well-thought-out and easy-to-use. Problems identified on these tests highlight areas that may need further definition by more formal and detailed tests.

The chapters on Recovery and Family Issues are positive and encouraging without being overly optimistic or excessively simplified, providing insight into problems that are new to most people unfamiliar with brain injury.

H. Terry Hutchison, M.D., Ph.D.
Associate Clinical Professor, Child Neurology
University of California, San Francisco, CA

■ In their book, *The Source for TBI – Children & Adolescents*, Drs. Lebby and Asbell have provided the reader with a truly useful, yet sophisticated and informative resource. The reader, whether a fully-trained professional, student, or interested parent, will find important, fascinating, and very useful information in this highly readable text. The information provided within this work is scientifically valid and based on current understanding of the effects of injury on the developing brain. The techniques discussed for assessment and treatment are well-established and evidence-based within the field of brain injury and recovery.

Drs. Lebby and Asbell have successfully integrated a wide range of highly-specialized information regarding brain development and function, along with the alterations in the behavioral expression of those functions that occur in children and adolescents as a result of a traumatic brain injury. They take the reader into the world of both language and non-language-based cognitive activities, with special emphasis on disruption of normal functioning resulting from brain trauma. Their efforts to illuminate this area of knowledge are made especially practical by their inclusion of evidence-based assessment and practice procedures to assist the professionals who work with a brain-injured population.

Errol F. Leifer, Ph.D., ABPP ABPN
Senior Neuropsychologist, Neuropsychology Department
Children's Hospital Central California, Madera, CA

■ Drs. Lebby and Asbell have co-authored a well-organized, current volume on traumatic brain injury and its sequelae in children and adolescents. The information provided within the text is well-founded within the current research regarding neurolinguistics. They provide a wealth of up-to-date information that teachers and clinicians will find useful and informative. The chapter on Language Disorders is exemplary, with its focus on practicality and its detailed examples of the various aphasia syndromes. This book is an excellent resource and will be a welcome addition to any clinician's library.

Carol Giovacchini, M.A., CCC-SLP
Speech-Language Pathologist
Children's Hospital Central California, Madera, CA

About the Authors

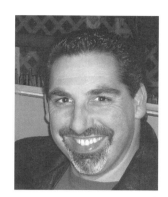

Paul C. Lebby, Ph.D., ABPS, received both his B.A. and his Ph.D. at the University of California Berkeley, with his studies being focused on human clinical neuroscience. His doctoral degree emphasized cognitive neuroscience and clinical neuropsychology. Dr. Lebby received his clinical training at the University of California San Francisco (UCSF) Medical Center where he completed several years of research, his pre-doctoral internship, and a post-doctoral fellowship within the Department of Neurology. He is board certified in forensic neuropsychology, and is frequently retained to give expert testimony regarding traumatic brain injury and recovery.

Currently, Dr. Lebby is on active medical staff at Children's Hospital Central California, in the Department of Medical Rehabilitation/Neuropsychology and at UCSF Medical Center in the Department of Neurology. Over the many years that Dr. Lebby has been in clinical practice, he has conducted thousands of evaluations on children and adolescents. He continues to be involved in clinical practice and in neurosurgical procedures where he maps brain functioning during brain surgery, assesses language lateralization via Wada (intracarotid sodium amytal) procedures, and acts as a consultant regarding brain injury and recovery.

Academically, Dr. Lebby is on the clinical faculty at Alliant International University where he is an associate professor. He has additional appointments as an assistant professor of neurology and assistant clinical professor of pediatrics at UCSF School of Medicine. Dr. Lebby has trained hundreds of students and continues to carry a teaching load in addition to his clinical duties. As part of his academic duties, he has chaired over 50 dissertations and supervises pre- and post-doctoral interns at his hospital practice. Dr. Lebby has multiple research publications and book chapters, and he continues to pursue an active research program. He lectures across the country on topics related to pediatric brain injury and recovery and presents each year at local and national conferences. He has a special interest in neuroimaging as it relates to pediatric brain injury and recovery and has developed new tests and techniques for assessing neurocognitive functioning in children and adolescents. Dr. Lebby's most important qualification, however, is his ability to explain difficult concepts relating to brain function and injury in a manner that is easily understood by all.

Shana J. Asbell, Ph.D., CCC-SLP, has been a clinical speech-language pathologist for over ten years and has recently earned a doctor of philosophy degree in clinical psychology with an emphasis in pediatric neuropsychology. Dr. Asbell's clinical experiences include working in a variety of organizations, including not-for-profit clinics, private practice, schools, and hospitals with children who present with a variety of neurodevelopmental, neurobehavioral, and neurocognitive disorders. She has provided assessment and therapeutic treatment for children ranging in age from preschool to young adulthood, as well as consultation to their families and other professionals regarding the speech-language and cognitive rehabilitation needs of neurologically-impaired children. Dr. Asbell has given presentations at ASHA and FLASHA and has presented workshops for professionals and parents. Currently, Dr. Asbell is a postdoctoral resident in neuropsychology at North Shore Children's Hospital in Salem, Massachusetts. She will complete her residency in clinical neuropsychology at Mary Free Bed Hospital in Grand Rapids, Michigan. This is Dr. Asbell's second publication with LinguiSystems. She is the co-author of *The Source for PDD: Assessment and Intervention* with Margaret Mapes Visconti.

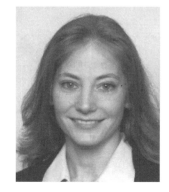

Dedications

We dedicate this book to our respective spouses, Kathy and Jeff, who patiently endured months of loss of the dining room tables to our computers and piles of work. We appreciate your tolerance of our seemingly endless hours of "book work." We are also grateful to our families and friends for their support and encouragement, and to those individuals with TBI whose lives and stories contributed to this work.

Edited by Karen Stontz • Page Layout by Lisa Parker • Cover Design and Illustrations by Jason Platt

Table of Contents

CD-ROM
- Lebby-Asbell Neurocognitive Screening Examination for Children (LANSE-C), Instructions, and Stimulus Book
- Lebby-Asbell Neurocognitive Screening Examination for Adolescents (LANSE-A), Instructions, and Stimulus Book
- Glasgow Coma Scale (GCS)
- Family Guide to The Rancho Levels of Cognitive Functioning

Introduction

The brain is a highly complex organ, making the effects of traumatic brain injury (TBI) in an individual difficult to predict. TBIs almost always affect some aspect of cognition. Sometimes damage causes disruption to primary abilities, such as language, memory, or visual and/or motor functioning. Other times, damage may result in more subtle impairments of cognition, such as arousal and attention, executive functioning, abstract reasoning, or thought processes.

Each child and adolescent who has sustained a brain injury presents with different deficits and follows a different course of recovery. Children with similar injuries do not experience identical deficits, and children with similar deficits may have different injuries. The overall similarities in impairment and recovery, however, tend to be greater than the individual differences.

It is crucial for a clinician working with this population to develop a general understanding of the effects a brain injury has on a child and his family. It is important to be aware of both the commonalities and the differences expected after a brain injury. *The Source for TBI – Children & Adolescents* presents the main aspects relating to brain injury in addition to the more subtle features that result from brain damage. This book also covers:

- brain anatomy and development
- TBI-related problems
- assessment procedures
- recovery processes
- recommendations for intervention
- family issues

We come from different specialty areas relating to the fields of neuroscience, brain injury, and language/communicative functioning. Both of us have years of experience assessing and treating children and adolescents with brain-related injuries. We also bring to this work many years of experience involving the research, study, and college-level teaching of the neurosciences and topics relating to brain injuries and dysfunction. While working together in a large children's hospital in central California, we had the opportunity to collaborate and produce *The Source for TBI – Children & Adolescents*. This book outlines the information and practice procedures that we have found to be useful and successful in the management of children and adolescents who have sustained TBIs.

We hope that you find *The Source for TBI – Children & Adolescents* helpful whether you work in a hospital, rehabilitation clinic, private practice office, or academic setting.

Paul and Shana

Interpreting Radiology Films

In clinical practice, radiology films are produced from the clinician's perspective (i.e., how the clinician views the patient). The clinician either faces a patient directly or interacts with a patient from the foot of the patient's hospital bed. As the clinician looks at the patient, the right hemisphere of the patient's brain is on the clinician's left side and the left hemisphere of the patient's brain is on the clinician's right side. Coronal and axial radiology images show the same view the clinician sees as he interacts with the patient. They appear to have the right and left sides reversed—the patient's left hemisphere is on the right side of the picture and his right hemisphere is on the left side of the picture.

We have flipped the brain scan images throughout *The Source for TBI – Children & Adolescents*. The right side of each picture within this text represents the right hemisphere and the left side of the picture represents the left hemisphere. This makes it easier for you to compare the pictures to the corresponding text because you do not need to mentally reverse the brain structures depicted.

Patient Information

The case examples cited throughout *The Source for TBI – Children & Adolescents* illustrate specific concepts or deficits related to TBI. These case examples represent actual patients whom we have treated; however, we have modified the names and ages to safeguard the confidentiality of our patients. Any correlation between a patient's name and/or injury and a known individual is purely coincidental. There are a few case examples in which the patients' real names and ages do appear. These patients have given us explicit permission to use their information within this book.

Glossary

Glossary terms are italicized and highlighted in purple throughout the text. The glossary is found on pages 217-222.

CD-ROM

The following assessments and tools are included on the enclosed CD-ROM.
- *Glasgow Coma Scale (GCS)*—This tool is used to measure acute brain injury. See pages 52-55 for more information regarding the *GCS*.
- *Lebby-Asbell Neurocognitive Screening Examination for Children (LANSE-C)* 6.0-11.11 years
  Lebby-Asbell Neurocognitive Screening Examination for Adolescents (LANSE-A) 12.0-17.11 years
  These screening examinations for children and adolescents were developed by the authors to assess basic neurocognitive functioning within a clinical practice. See pages 138-148 for more information regarding the *LANSE-C* and the *LANSE-A*.
- Instructions and Stimulus Books for the *LANSE-C* and the *LANSE-A*
- *Family Guide to The Rancho Levels of Cognitive Functioning*—This classification scale describes the behaviors a patient may exhibit during the stages of recovery after a brain injury. See pages 154-159 for more information regarding the *The Rancho Los Amigos Levels of Cognitive Functioning (RLA)*.

Chapter 1

Functional Brain Anatomy

The relationship between brain function and behavior has been studied for centuries, but it was not until recently that attention has been given to the effects of brain injury on a child's development and functioning. Brain injury in children, which is the focus of this book, is still a relatively new field of study that continues to change rapidly.

Working with children and adults who have a traumatic brain injury (TBI) can be very rewarding; however, many clinicians may feel poorly equipped to assess and treat persons with TBI because of their limited educational background in neuroanatomy. The complexities relating to brain injury can seem overwhelming, but a basic understanding of neuroanatomy will help you identify and interpret problems caused by a brain injury. (See Appendix 1A, pages 24-25, for a brief historical review of functional neuroanatomy.)

▌ Anatomy of the Brain

The human nervous system is divided into the central and peripheral nervous systems. The *central nervous system* (CNS) consists of the brain and the spinal cord and plays a key role in controlling behavior. The *peripheral nervous system* (PNS) is made up of all the neurons in the body outside of the central nervous system.

The PNS includes 12 pairs of *cranial nerves* that connect the brain with the body but do not pass through the spinal cord. There are motor and sensory cranial nerves and some nerves that have both functions. The cranial nerves allow for functions such as movement of the face, eye, and neck muscles; facial sensations; swallowing; smell; vision; and hearing. They also allow for modulation of bodily functions involving the heart, lungs, and gastrointestinal tract. (See Appendix 1B, pages 26-27, for more detailed information regarding these nerves.)

The PNS is further divided into the *somatic nervous system* and the *autonomic nervous system*. These systems work together to allow information to be sent between the spinal cord and the body and to regulate bodily states. The somatic nervous system is made up of two types of neurons—afferent neurons, which carry sensory information from the sense organs toward the central nervous system, and efferent neurons, which carry motor instructions to the muscles. The autonomic nervous system works to maintain normal internal functions by regulating the many organs, muscles, and glands within the body.

The branch of anatomy that studies the organization of the nervous system is called *neuroanatomy*. Neuroanatomy can be divided into two areas—microanatomy and macroanatomy.

Microanatomy

Microanatomy involves the study of brain structures at a microscopic level and relates to *neurons* and *glia*, two types of cells that help to form the brain.

Neurons are found in every area of the brain and spinal cord and compose the CNS and PNS. They are specialized nerve cells that can react to stimuli and transmit impulses. Neurons communicate information within the brain and between the brain and the body. They also communicate with each other using specialized chemicals called *neurotransmitters*. These chemicals flow from one cell to another across very small gaps called *synapses*.

A neuron consists of a soma (the body of the cell that contains the nucleus), dendrites, and an axon. *Dendrites*, which are short branches that extend from the body of the cell, bring information into the cell. The *axon* is a long outgrowth that carries information out of the cell to the next neuron.

Axons connect the areas of the brain. Some axons connect different areas of the *cortex* to allow for integrated brain functioning. These fiber pathways are critical for normal brain activity. Disruption of communication due to TBI-related axonal damage can result in significant deficits. Other axons connect the various structures of the brain with the body via the spinal cord or cranial nerves to allow for motor and sensory functioning.

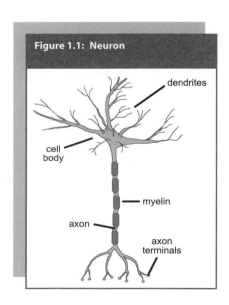

Figure 1.1: Neuron

Glial cells hold brain tissue together and perform general housekeeping functions, such as assisting in the repair of damaged tissue; regulating the flow of substances like proteins and ions; and producing *myelin*, the fatty substance that surrounds axons.

Macroanatomy

Macroanatomy relates to the study of the larger brain structures that make up the central nervous system. The brain can be divided into areas based on cellular structure and function. The largest division is between the right and left hemispheres. Other divisions are not as easy to identify but involve the four lobes of the brain's cortex (frontal, parietal, temporal, and occipital), the deeper subcortical structures, and the cerebellum.

❚ Brain Areas Based on Cellular Structure

Neurons and glial cells are not the only cells that make up brain tissue. On the contrary, there are many structures and substances in the brain that are made from other types of cells, tissue, or fluid. These include meninges, cerebral spinal fluid, ventricles, blood, and blood vessels.

▶ Meninges

Beneath the protective hard bone of the skull are meninges, the system of membranes that envelop the central nervous system. The primary functions of the meninges are to protect and nourish the brain and the spinal cord. Meninges are made up of three layers of skin—the dura mater, the arachnoid layer, and the pia mater.

- Just beneath the skull is a thick layer of tissue called the ***dura mater*** or *dura*. The dura mater surrounds the brain and separates the right and left hemispheres (***falx cerebri***) and the lower part of the brain from the upper cerebral hemispheres (***tentorium cerebelli***). Cavities in the dura, called ***venous sinuses***, allow blood to flow out of the brain.

- Beneath the dura is the ***arachnoid layer***, a hollow, web-like layer filled with cerebral spinal fluid. This layer contains ***arachnoid granulations*** that reabsorb cerebral spinal fluid and allow the fluid to exit the brain and re-enter the blood supply via the venous sinuses.

- The ***pia mater*** is between the arachnoid layer and the surface of the cortex. Pia mater is a delicate layer of tissue that covers the entire surface of the brain. It contains a matrix of tiny blood vessels that supplies the surface of the cortex. This layer also forms the choroid plexus, which produces cerebral spinal fluid.

▶ Cerebral Spinal Fluid and Ventricles

The brain floats in ***cerebral spinal fluid*** (CSF). CSF contains a reservoir of hormones and nutrients for the central nervous system. It also cushions the brain and protects it from small shocks and jolts that are caused by minor bumps or normal movement of the head.

The ***choroid plexus*** is found in several large, hollow spaces within the brain called ***ventricles***. It makes approximately 500 milliliters of CSF from blood plasma each day—about the same amount of fluid as contained in a 16-ounce water bottle. Most CSF is made in the ***lateral ventricles***, the large cavities situated in the right and left hemispheres. The CSF that fills these ventricles provides additional protection for the brain.

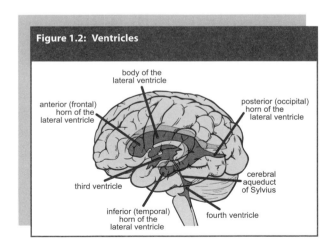

Figure 1.2: Ventricles

body of the lateral ventricle

anterior (frontal) horn of the lateral ventricle

posterior (occipital) horn of the lateral ventricle

third ventricle

cerebral aqueduct of Sylvius

inferior (temporal) horn of the lateral ventricle

fourth ventricle

CSF flows under pressure down from the lateral ventricles to the *third ventricle* located in the center of the brain. From the third ventricle, the fluid flows down a small, tube-like structure, called the *cerebral aqueduct of Sylvius*, to the *fourth ventricle*. Eventually the CSF flows to the outside of the brain and spinal cord into the arachnoid layer and to various other cavities within the brain called *cisterns*. CSF in the arachnoid layer supports the brain and spinal cord structures. It is then reabsorbed back into the venous blood supply through the arachnoid granulations in the second layer of the meninges.

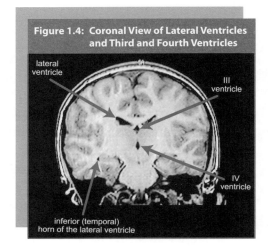

Figure 1.3: Sagittal View of Right Lateral Ventricle and Fourth Ventricle

right lateral ventricle

IV ventricle

▶ Blood Vessels

Blood vessels in the brain are constructed differently than other blood vessels within the body. They are designed to protect the brain from toxic chemicals and substances. The vessels have smaller gaps between the cells which make a barrier between the blood and the brain known as the *blood-brain barrier*.

Figure 1.4: Coronal View of Lateral Ventricles and Third and Fourth Ventricles

lateral ventricle

III ventricle

IV ventricle

inferior (temporal) horn of the lateral ventricle

Brain cells need a large supply of energy in the form of oxygen and glucose. To meet this need, the brain contains numerous blood vessels that carry approximately three-fourths of a liter of oxygenated blood to the brain every minute. Four main blood vessels supply the brain—the right and left *internal carotid arteries* and the right and left *vertebral arteries*.

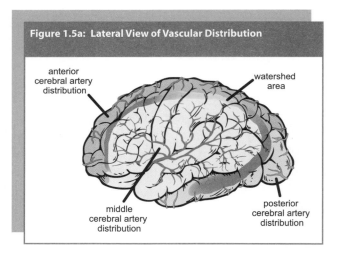

Figure 1.5a: Lateral View of Vascular Distribution

anterior cerebral artery distribution

watershed area

middle cerebral artery distribution

posterior cerebral artery distribution

- Blood flows from the internal carotid arteries to the right and left middle cerebral arteries which travel to the outside edges of the brain and supply the frontal lobes, parietal lobes, and most of the temporal lobes. The middle cerebral arteries also send branches to the deeper, sub-cortical structures of the thalamus, hypothalamus, basal ganglia, and limbic system. Blood from the carotid arteries also flows to the right and left anterior cerebral arteries, which supply the inner or medial surfaces of the brain between the two hemispheres.

- Blood flows from the vertebral arteries into a single vessel called the *basilar artery*. The blood flows from the basilar artery through the right and left posterior cerebral arteries to the occipital lobes at the back of the cortex and to the underside of the temporal lobes. Blood also flows from the basilar artery via smaller vessels to the hindbrain, brain stem, cerebellum, and spinal cord.

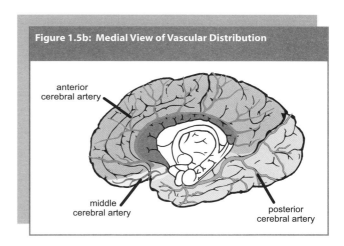

Figure 1.5b: Medial View of Vascular Distribution

anterior cerebral artery

middle cerebral artery

posterior cerebral artery

- Blood exits the brain by draining into several veins, which, in turn, drain into the cavernous sinus and venous sinuses in the dura mater. Eventually the blood leaves the brain via the *internal jugular veins*.

The *watershed area* is located between the fingers of the middle, anterior, and posterior cerebral arteries. The middle cerebral arteries do not cover the entire lateral surface of the brain. The edges of the lateral surface receive blood from the anterior cerebral artery at the front and the posterior cerebral artery at the back. This leaves the watershed area with poor arterial coverage and blood perfusion, so problems with blood supply are likely to result in damage to this region.

The *circle of Willis* is where blood vessels that originate from the carotid and vertebral arteries and from the right and left hemispheres become combined in a circle-like vascular structure called an *anastomosis*. In a healthy brain, not much blood flows through the communicating arteries due to equal blood pressure on each side of these connecting vessels, but when there is brain damage or disrupted blood flow, the circle of Willis allows blood from healthy areas or vessels to be transported to the damaged areas.

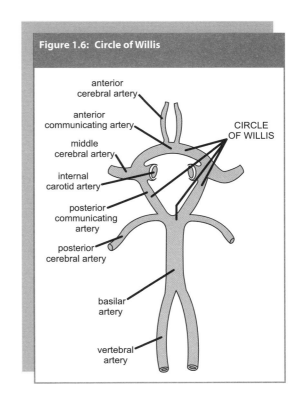

Figure 1.6: Circle of Willis

anterior cerebral artery

anterior communicating artery

middle cerebral artery

internal carotid artery

posterior communicating artery

posterior cerebral artery

CIRCLE OF WILLIS

basilar artery

vertebral artery

Functional Areas of the Brain

There are three basic areas of the brain—the forebrain, the midbrain, and the hindbrain. Each of these areas consists of smaller brain structures as shown in the chart below.

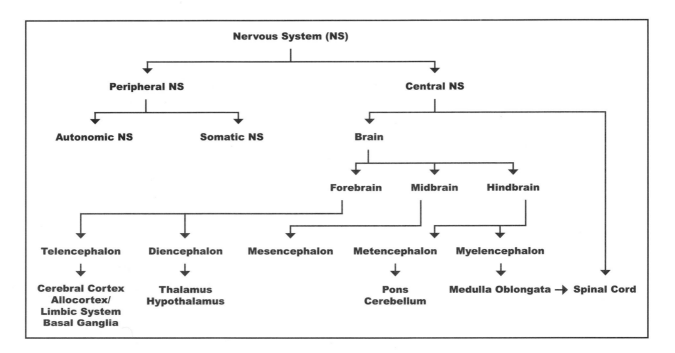

- A glossary of anatomical terms relating to the brain and spinal cord is included in Appendix 1C on page 28.
- For a summary of the parts of the brain and their general functions, see Appendix 1D on page 29.
- To view sagittal, coronal, and axial cuts of the brain, see Appendix 1E on page 30.

▸ Forebrain

The forebrain consists of two parts—the telencephalon and the diencephalon.

Telencephalon

The *telencephalon*, also known as the cerebrum, is the part of the brain that allows us to use intellect and social skills, control our emotions, process sensory information, and control voluntary movements. The telencephalon consists of the cerebral cortex; the allocortex/limbic system, including the hippocampi and the mammillary bodies; and the basal ganglia. The cerebral cortex is divided into four main areas—the frontal lobes, the parietal lobes, the temporal lobes, and the occipital lobes.

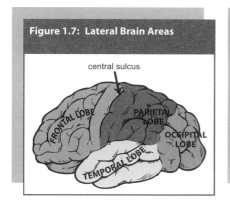

Figure 1.7: Lateral Brain Areas

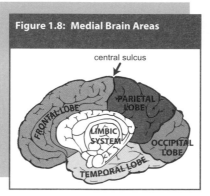

Figure 1.8: Medial Brain Areas

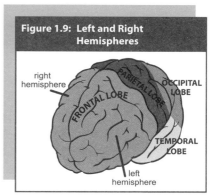

Figure 1.9: Left and Right Hemispheres

■ Cerebral Cortex

The cerebral cortex forms the outer layer of the brain and is divided into the left and right hemispheres. Most cognitive functions take place in the cortex. In the majority of people, the left hemisphere controls language functioning while the right hemisphere controls more non-language-based skills which require visual-spatial processing. Each hemisphere has a frontal, parietal, temporal, and occipital lobe.

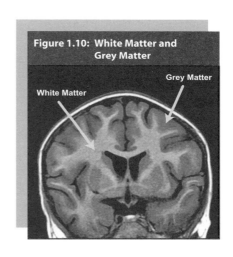

Figure 1.10: White Matter and Grey Matter

The cortex resembles the bark of a tree—bumpy and wrinkled with many grooves known as *sulci* that separate elevated bulges called *gyri*. The cortex is commonly called *grey matter* because it is made up of neurons which are dark in color.

The layer below the grey matter consists of the communication fibers. This layer is known as *white matter* because of the white appearance of myelin, the fatty substance surrounding the fibers. The communication fibers connect areas of the cortex with other areas of cortex and with deeper structures within the brain. They also connect brain structures with the body via the spinal cord and the cranial nerves.

Communication Fibers	Connections
corpus callosum	connects the right and left hemispheres
corona radiata	connects the cortex with the deeper brain structures
internal capsule	connects the cortex with the spinal cord
optic tract/radiations	transmits visual information from the eyes to the cortex
arcuate fasciculus	connects posterior language areas to frontal speech areas (Wernicke's area to Broca's area)
uncinate fasciculus	connects the frontal lobe to the limbic structures
longitudinal fasciculus	connects the frontal areas to the parietal areas

The Four Lobes of the Cortex:

1. Frontal Lobes

The *frontal lobes* are located in the front of each hemisphere. The general role of the frontal lobes is to allow a person to function in an intellectually and socially complex environment. Specific functions include the ability to learn and store knowledge; to reason using visual and language-based information; to use intellectual, social, emotional, and executive functioning skills; and to provide for voluntary motor control and the motor output for speech. The part of the frontal lobes closest to the center of the brain works with the allocortex/limbic system to control primitive drives, such as aggression and rage, sexual behavior, predation, and fear.

The frontal lobes have four areas relating to motor output—the primary motor cortex, the premotor cortex, the frontal eye fields, and Broca's area.

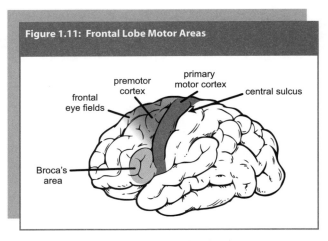

Figure 1.11: Frontal Lobe Motor Areas

The *primary motor cortex* is located at the back of the frontal lobes and is aligned almost vertically. At the top, it folds between the left and right hemispheres. It controls the motor functions of the face, arms, torso, lower body, and legs.

The *premotor cortex*, or *secondary motor cortex* is located in front of the primary motor cortex. It is used for complex motor functions, such as motor planning and the initiation of skilled motor sequences.

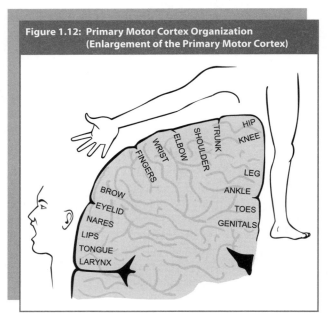

Figure 1.12: Primary Motor Cortex Organization (Enlargement of the Primary Motor Cortex)

The *frontal eye fields* are in front of the premotor cortex, close to the front of the brain. This area receives input from the visual and auditory environment. The frontal eye fields organize head and eye movements and gaze shifts.

Broca's area is located just in front and at the bottom of the primary motor cortex. This area is responsible for the motor output of expressive speech.

The *central sulcus* is a fold in the cerebral cortex that separates the frontal lobes from the parietal lobes, thereby separating the motor and sensory areas of the brain.

2. Parietal Lobes

The *parietal lobes* are located directly behind the frontal lobes. These lobes are sometimes called *multi-modal cortices* because they are involved in:

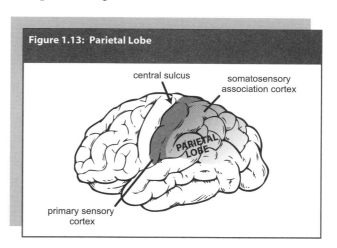

Figure 1.13: Parietal Lobe

- processing language and visual, tactile, and auditory information
- integrating sensory information
- interpreting and understanding information relating to self, others, and the environment
- identifying objects
- understanding spatial relationships relating to the body
- interpreting pain and touch

The parietal lobes are divided into two areas—the primary sensory cortex and the somatosensory association cortex.

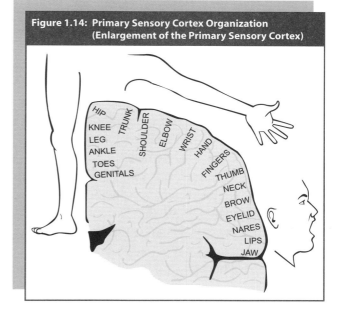

Figure 1.14: Primary Sensory Cortex Organization (Enlargement of the Primary Sensory Cortex)

The *primary sensory cortex* is a narrow strip of tissue that extends from one side of the cortex near the ear over the top of the brain. It receives sensory input from the body and mediates our sense of touch. The bottom of the primary cortex strip receives input from the face, the middle of the strip receives input from the arms and torso, and the top of the strip receives input from the lower torso and legs.

Behind the primary sensory cortex is an area called the *somatosensory association cortex*. This part of the parietal lobe integrates information from the various senses, such as touch, vision, and auditory information.

3. Temporal Lobes

The *temporal lobes* lie at the sides of the brain just beneath the frontal and parietal lobes. They are involved in auditory processing, language semantics, emotion, and memory formation/retrieval. The temporal lobes contain the following areas.

- The *primary auditory cortex* allows us to perceive sound.

- The *auditory association cortex* helps us to recognize sounds.

- *Wernicke's area* allows us to understand and use language to communicate. It is located in an area that extends from the temporal lobe to the parietal lobe (temporal-parietal region).

The temporal lobes also have deeper structures within the brain that are involved with memory and emotion.

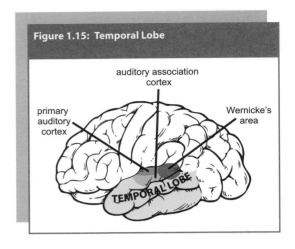

Figure 1.15: Temporal Lobe

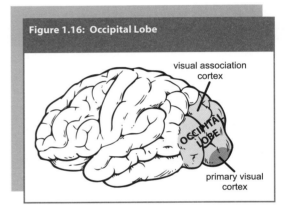

Figure 1.16: Occipital Lobe

4. Occipital Lobes

The *occipital lobes*, the smallest of the four lobes of the brain, are located at the back of the brain, just behind the parietal lobes. They receive and process visual information.

The occipital lobes contain the primary visual cortex and the visual association cortex. The *primary visual cortex* receives basic visual information relating to contrast and to orientation of lines, color, and movement. It then relays this information to the secondary and tertiary visual cortices, also known as the *visual association cortex*. The visual association cortex processes the information at increasing levels of complexity and allows us to see intricate scenes and to identify and make sense of the things we see.

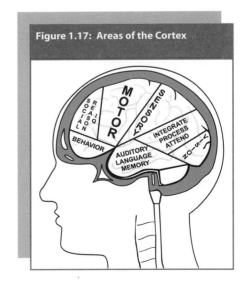

Figure 1.17: Areas of the Cortex

■ Allocortex/Limbic System

The allocortex is also called the *limbic system* or *Papez circuit*. It sits below the main part of the cortex, deep within the brain. The limbic structures control basic functions that are sometimes thought of as being primitive and relate to behaviors such as:

- emotion (e.g., aggression, sexual behavior, predation)

- motor and visceral responses that initiate approach or avoidance behaviors (i.e., during fighting or mating)

- expression of rage or fear

- instinctive and species specific behaviors (e.g., dominance-submission)

- storage and retrieval of memories

- pleasure and reinforcement

The allocortex is tightly connected to the frontal lobes of the cortex. The communication fibers of the uncinate fasciculus allow the frontal lobes to keep the primitive emotions and drives associated with the limbic system "in check" (e.g., aggression, rage, sexual behavior, predation, and fear), thus giving people the ability to behave appropriately in various social situations.

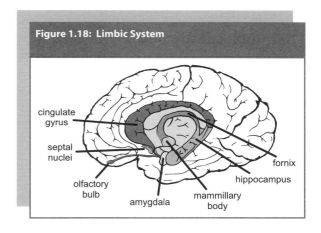

Figure 1.18: Limbic System

cingulate gyrus
septal nuclei
olfactory bulb
amygdala
fornix
hippocampus
mammillary body

Hippocampi
The *hippocampi* are part of the allocortex/limbic system and are located deep in the temporal lobes. The hippocampi are highly involved with memory functioning of the brain and are responsible for transferring information to and from the cortex where memories are stored. They are also involved with emotional functioning and are connected to other limbic structures by extensive neural pathways.

Amygdala
The *amygdala nuclei* are connected to all areas of the brain and are involved with instinctive fear responses and the control of the hypothalamic-midbrain mechanisms of aggression and defensive behavior. The amygdala also contain receptors for estrogen and androgens, such as testosterone, allowing for hormonal control of behavior.

Mammillary Bodies

The *mammillary bodies* are two groups of nuclei within the limbic system that play a role in emotion and memory. They are connected to the hippocampi by a bundle of fibers called the *fornix*. The mammillary bodies are also connected to the thalamus via the mammillo-thalamic tract, allowing for integration of information between the thalamus and other limbic structures.

Septal Nuclei

The *septal nuclei* are located just anterior and inferior to the corpus callosum. They have a modulatory role involving emotions. Damage to different nuclei within the septal region can produce extremes of emotion, from rage and uncontrolled aggression to euphoria and pleasurable feelings. The septal region also exerts control over sympathetic (arousal) and parasympathetic (relaxation) nervous system functioning.

Cingulate Gyrus

The *cingulate gyrus* connects the areas of the limbic system, such as the hippocampus, amygdala, and prefrontal cortex. Control from the prefrontal cortex via the cingulate gyrus allows a child to modulate emotional responses in order to function in a complex social environment. The cingulate gyrus is also involved in the integration of sensory information with emotional responses, the modulation of emotional responses to pain, and the regulation of aggression.

Fornix

The *fornix* is the major pathway that connects structures within the limbic system. The fornix begins at the dorsal end of the hippocampi, encircles the dorsal thalamus, and comes to an end at the mammillary bodies.

Olfactory Bulbs

The *olfactory bulbs* are located on the underside of the anterior-most part of the brain. They allow us to perceive and discriminate odors, providing our sense of smell. The olfactory bulbs connect directly to the limbic system via the amygdala and deeper nuclei in the basal forebrain. The direct links between the olfactory bulbs and the limbic system account for the strong connections between smells and emotions.

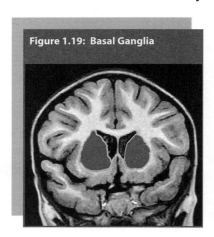

Figure 1.19: Basal Ganglia

■ Basal Ganglia

The basal ganglia are groups of nuclei, or cell bodies, deep in the brain. There are two sets of basal ganglia, mirrored in the left and right hemispheres.

The primary function of the basal ganglia is to modulate the body's motor system so that a person can make smooth, controlled movements. The basal ganglia are also involved in the automaticity of functions, routines, and behaviors. For example, when we first learn a skill (e.g., playing the piano, driving a car, riding a bicycle), we must use our cortex to think about what we are doing. As the skill becomes automatic, we begin to rely more on the basal ganglia structures. Eventually the basal ganglia may take over the functions so that we do not have to think as much about doing the skill. It becomes automatic.

Diencephalon

The *diencephalon* includes the thalamus and the hypothalamus.

The *thalamus* is a large, dual-lobed mass of grey matter cells located near the top of the brain stem. It can be thought of as a relay station for information that goes in and out of the cortex. Pathways through the thalamus connect with different areas of the frontal, parietal, temporal, and occipital lobes.

The thalamus also processes sensory information, deciding what information is important and what can be ignored. For example, when you first put on clothing, you feel it against your skin, but after a few minutes you no longer notice it. Even though the sensory signals from your skin are still arriving at the brain, the thalamus has stopped sending them to the cortex because the signals are not important to functioning.

The *hypothalamus* is located below the thalamus at the base of the brain. It is composed of many different nuclei, or groups of cells. The nuclei control internal bodily states, the autonomic nervous system, and the hormonal system via the pituitary gland. Although the hypothalamus is only the size of a pea and takes up less than one percent of the brain, it regulates some very important functions, such as:

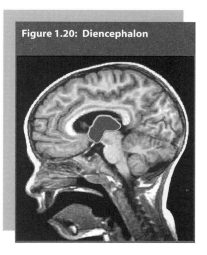

Figure 1.20: Diencephalon

- emotion
- hunger
- thirst
- body temperature
- sexual/reproductive behavior
- circadian rhythms (changes in mental and physical characteristics that occur during the course of a day)
- the fight-or-flight response (rapid heartbeat, fast breathing, widening of the pupils, and increased blood flow caused by fear or excitement)
- autonomic responses to environmental stimuli, such as pain

Mesencephalon

The *mesencephalon*, or midbrain, is located directly below the diencephalon. It contains nuclei and pathways that control movement, arousal, sleep, attention, muscle tone, pain, and species typical behaviors (e.g., mating, fighting), as well as areas that control visual and auditory responses.

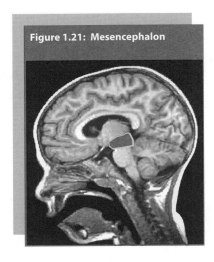

Figure 1.21: Mesencephalon

▸ Hindbrain

The hindbrain is located below the midbrain. It consists of two parts—the metencephalon and the myelencephalon, or brain stem. The parts of the hindbrain function collectively to support vital bodily processes, such as the coordination of motor activity, posture, equilibrium, sleep patterns, and the regulation of unconscious but essential functions, such as breathing and blood circulation.

Metencephalon

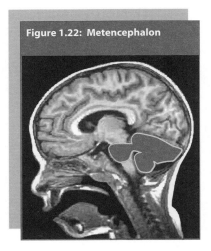

Figure 1.22: Metencephalon

The *metencephalon* includes the pons and the cerebellum.

The *pons* is located on the anterior portion of the metencephalon, an area where many pathways pass in and out of the brain. The pons receives information from visual areas to control eye and facial movements and plays a role in controlling sleep patterns and central nervous system arousal.

The *cerebellum* is located behind the pons on the underside of the brain. It looks like a small brain. It has grey and white matter, a cortex, and it is bumpy on the outside with sulci and gyri.

The cerebellum plays an important role in the integration of sensory perception and motor output. It is primarily involved with the coordination of movements, balance, muscle tone, posture, and equilibrium. Nuclei in the cerebellum receive input from the visual, auditory, vestibular, and somatosensory systems. The cerebellum integrates and modifies the motor output accordingly.

The cerebellum also modulates the activity of many areas of the brain involved with cognitive functioning. Cerebellar activity has been related to numerous cognitive abilities, including attention, language, memory, social awareness, and intellect.

The Source for TBI – Children & Adolescents   22

Myelencephalon (Brain Stem)

The *myelencephalon* includes the medulla oblongata and the spinal cord. It is involved with many basic functions, including the following.

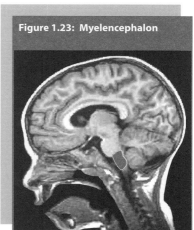

Figure 1.23: Myelencephalon

- movements of the eyes and mouth
- relaying sensory messages related to temperature, pain, and hunger
- respiration
- consciousness
- cardiac function
- body temperature regulation
- involuntary muscle movements
- sneezing
- coughing
- vomiting
- swallowing

The *medulla oblongata*, often called *medulla*, is the lower portion of the brain stem. It is the most vital part of the entire brain and contains important control centers for the heart and lungs. The medulla has four main functions.

- It connects the brain with the spinal cord.

- It contains the *reticular nuclei*, which control the heartbeat, breathing, and muscle tone.

- It sends input to the face, mouth, throat, and eyes.

- It relays information from the spinal cord to the thalamus and motor information from the brain to the spinal cord.

▶ Spinal Cord

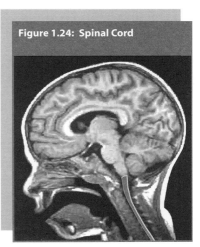

Figure 1.24: Spinal Cord

The *spinal cord* can be considered an extension of the medulla oblongata. The spinal cord is composed of a large bundle of nerve fibers that extends from the base of the brain to the lower back. It carries messages to and from the brain and the rest of the body. The spinal cord is similar in composition to the brain, in that it contains brain cells (grey matter), pathways (white matter), dura, arachnoid layers, pia, and cerebral spinal fluid.

Evidence found on an Egyptian papyrus scroll dated 1700 B.C. cites how a head injury caused peripheral dysfunction. In the fifth century B.C., Hippocrates noted that disorders of the brain could lead to altered mental status. Despite these early studies of the brain, it wasn't until the last 200 years that a clear, scientific understanding of the relationship between brain functioning and behavior was formulated. In the last 100 years, military studies of adults injured during war have significantly increased this understanding. Some of the most notable advances in understanding brain-behavior relationships have come from scientists who studied the anatomy and structure of the brain. Their research is of particular interest to clinicians who work with individuals who have a traumatic brain injury.

▶ **Franz Joseph Gall** (1758-1828)

Gall, who is regarded as the father of *phrenology*, is considered to be the first scientist to systematically study each part of the brain to determine its function. He identified the areas of the brain responsible for many behaviors, including language. Gall studied the shape of the skull and its relationship to functional abilities. He hypothesized that the shape of the skull was related to the size of the brain structures. His theory was that the brain would be larger in areas where a person was most proficient. This was the beginning of the scientific study leading to functional neuroanatomy.

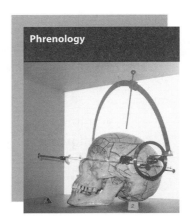

Phrenology

▶ **Paul Broca** (1824-1880)

Broca is one of the best-known scientists in the field of brain localization. In the late 1800s, he published articles demonstrating the existence of a speech center in the brain and defined an organic basis for aphasia. This research formed the neurological basis for Broca's aphasia.

Although Broca's discoveries disproved Gall's basic premise of phrenology (i.e., the surface of the skull does not reflect the topography of the brain), they validated Gall's theory that specific areas in the brain are responsible for specific brain functions. (See Chapter 4, pages 71-73, for more information on Broca's aphasia.)

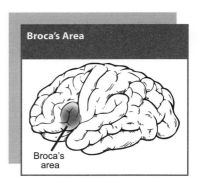

Broca's Area

Broca's area

▶ **Karl Wernicke** (1848-1904)

Wernicke is best known for his work on sensory aphasia. His interest in psychiatry led him to study anatomy and neuropathology of the brain. In the late 1800s, he published information on aphasia that contained precise analysis of anatomical damage with comparison to the clinical behaviors he saw in his patients. His research led to the discovery of what is now called Wernicke's aphasia. (See Chapter 4, pages 73-74, for more information on Wernicke's aphasia.)

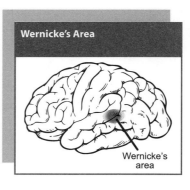

Wernicke's Area

Wernicke's area

▶ **Korbinian Brodmann** (1868-1918)

In 1909, Brodmann identified 52 discrete areas of the cortex in which the cellular structures were clearly differentiated from other areas. He diagrammed the areas on a picture of the brain based on the cytoarchitecture (shape and organization) of cells and the cells' staining properties. Later, the areas identified by Brodmann were found to generally correlate with functional regions of the brain. We now know that the cortex is divided into discrete areas with different cellular structures and organization, and these areas provide different functions for the brain.

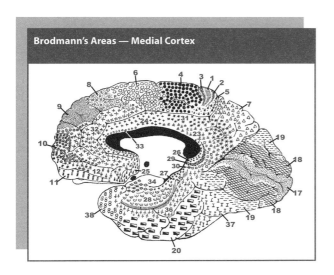
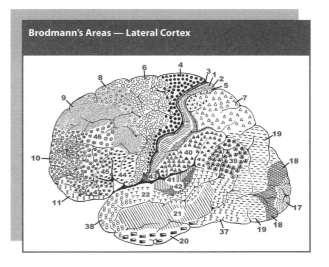

Key to Brodmann's Areas

Areas 1, 2, 3	Primary Somatosensory Cortex		Areas 26, 30	Retrosplenial Cortex
Area 4	Primary Motor Cortex		Area 27	Amygdala – Medial Temporal Lobe
Area 5	Somatosensory Association Cortex		Areas 28, 34	Entorhinal Cortex – Medial Temporal Lobe
Area 6	Supplementary/Pre-Motor Cortex		Area 35	Perirhinal Cortex – Medial Temporal Lobe
Area 7	Somatosensory Association Cortex Pre-cuneus		Area 36	Parahippocampal Cortex – Medial Temporal Lobe
Area 8	Frontal Eye Fields		Area 37	Fusiform Gyrus
Areas 9, 46	Dorsolateral Frontal Cortex		Area 39	Area close to the Angular Gyrus
Area 10	Frontal Pole		Area 40	Supramarginal Gyrus
Areas 11, 12	Orbital-Frontal Lobe		Area 41	Superior Temporal Gyrus – Primary Auditory Cortex
Areas 13, 14	Insular Cortex		Area 42	Superior Temporal Gyrus – Secondary Auditory Association Cortex
Areas 15, 38	Anterior Temporal Lobe			
Area 16	Insular – Association Cortex		Area 43	Subcentral Area (at base of somatosensory gyrus)
Area 17	Primary Visual Cortex (VI)		Area 44	Subfrontal Pars Opercularis (Broca's area)
Area 18	Secondary Visual Association Cortex (V2)		Area 45	Subfrontal Pars Triangularis
Area 19	Tertiary Visual Association Cortex (V3)		Area 47	Inferior Orbital Frontal Gyrus
Area 20	Temporal Lobe – Inferior Gyrus		Area 48	Retrosubicular Area of the Temporal Lobe
Area 21	Temporal Lobe – Middle Gyrus		Area 49	Parasubicular Area (between presubiculum and entorhinal cortex)
Area 22	Temporal Lobe – Superior Gyrus (close to Wernicke's Area)			
			Area 50	Band of cortex located on the fronto-parietal operculum
Areas 23, 24, 29, 31, 32, 33	Cingulate Gyrus		Area 51	Piriform and the periamygdaloid cortices
Area 25	Subgenual Cortex		Area 52	Parainsular Area (between temporal lobe and insular)

Note: Not all areas are visible in the pictures, and not all areas are present in humans. The areas were mapped based on the cytoarchitecture of the cells (cell structure, organization, and staining properties), and not on function. Therefore, there is not an exact mapping between all of the numbered areas and functional regions, such as Wernicke's area or the angular gyrus.

The following chart lists the 12 cranial nerves, their functions, and the way(s) you can clinically assess the functioning of each nerve.

Cranial Nerve	Type of Nerve	Function	Clinical Assessment
I. Olfactory	sensory	sense of smell	• Have the patient close his eyes. Then hold something (e.g., orange, peanut butter) under his nose and ask him to identify the smell.
II. Optic	sensory	sense of vision	• Have the patient read fine print with a small font or use an eye chart to test near and far vision. • Test visual fields by placing an object in the patient's right or left visual field. Test each eye separately, then both eyes together.
III. Oculomotor	motor	external eye muscles	• Look for drooping of the patient's eyelids (*ptosis*).
		pupil size	• Check for normal pupil size. Check each eye separately, then both eyes together.
		accommodation	• Move a pen close to the nose to check accommodation (eyes converge, lenses focus/thicken, pupils constrict).
		eye movements	• Observe for limited eye movement and jerky eye movement (*nystagmus*).
IV. Trochlear	motor	eye movements	• Have the patient follow your finger without moving his head (up/down, left/right, diagonally). • Observe for limited eye movement and jerky eye movement (*nystagmus*).
V. Trigeminal	motor and sensory	facial sensation (three branches—opthalmic, maxillary, mandibular)	• Have the patient close his eyes. Then touch his face and ask him to identify where you touched him.
		chewing movements	• Ask the patient to attempt to move his jaw as you apply opposing force.
VI. Abducens	motor	lateral eye movements	• Ask the patient to track side-to-side by following your finger. Test each eye separately, then both eyes together. • Observe for limited eye movement and nystagmus.
VII. Facial	motor and sensory	facial expressions	• Observe the patient's smile, wrinkled forehead, winks of each eye, and puffed cheeks. • Look for asymmetry with facial expressions.

Cranial Nerve	Type of Nerve	Function	Clinical Assessment
(Facial, *cont.*)		identification of taste	• Ask the patient to identify different tastes.
VIII. Auditory-vestibulocochlear	sensory	identification of sounds, hearing	• Have the patient close his eyes. Then test his hearing by rubbing two of your fingers together close to one of his ears. Ask the patient to identify which ear your fingers are next to. Test each ear separately, then both ears together.
		balance and equilibrium	• Have the patient touch his nose and then touch your finger. • Observe the patient as he stands with his feet together and eyes closed. Stand close to him in case he begins to sway or fall. • Look for smooth, coordinated movements or swaying when the patient is standing with his eyes closed.
IX. Glossopharyngeal	motor and sensory	taste and other sensations of the tongue	• Observe the patient as he says, "Ah."
		movements used for swallowing	• Watch the patient swallow.
X. Vagus	motor and sensory	gag reflex	• Have the patient protrude his tongue. Then touch the back of his throat with a tongue depressor to observe his gag reflex.
		modulation of the functioning of the pharnyx, larynx, heart, lungs, palate, trachea, gastrointestinal tract, and external ear	• Base assessment on the presence of specific symptoms.
XI. Accessory	motor	shoulder and head movements	• Observe the patient's ability to shrug his shoulders and turn his head against resistance. • Look for weakness.
XII. Hypoglossal	motor	tongue movements	• Have the patient protrude his tongue, move his tongue rapidly from side-to-side, and push his tongue against resistance. • Look to make sure the patient's tongue protrudes along the midline and has normal strength.

▶ **Terms Related to Neurons (Nerve Cells)**

column	a set of neurons organized perpendicular to the cortical surface
tract	a pathway or projection from one area to another in the brain
nerve	a collection of neurons in the periphery that connect the CNS with the body
nucleus	a group of neuron cell bodies within the CNS
ganglion	a group of neuron cell bodies outside of the CNS (except the basal ganglia)

▶ **Terms Related to the Brain and Spinal Cord (CNS) When Dealing with the Human Body**

superior	toward the head
inferior	toward the feet
anterior	in front
posterior	behind
ventral	toward the abdomen – front of the body
dorsal	along the back of the body

▶ **Directional Terms for Discussing the Human Brain**

rostral	toward the nose
caudal	toward the tail
superior	toward the top of the head
inferior	toward the base of the skull
anterior	toward the frontal poles (front of brain)
posterior	toward the occipital poles (back of brain)
lateral	away from the neuraxis (center of the CNS)
medial	toward the neuraxis (center of the CNS)

▶ **Directional Terms for Discussing the Human Brain Stem and Spinal Cord**

transverse	across the brain stem or spinal cord
longitudinal	running up and down the brain stem or spinal cord

▶ **Terms Regarding the Direction of Nerve Fibers**

ascending	from the spinal cord to the brain (sensory)
descending	from the brain to the spinal cord (motor)
ipsilateral	the same side of the brain and body
contralateral	the opposite side of the brain and body
decussate	where the fibers cross to the opposite side of the body

▶ **Frontal Lobes**
- intellect and reasoning
- socially appropriate judgment and insight
- behavioral and emotional control
- executive functioning
- expressive speech (usually left hemisphere)
- prosody and use of intonation (usually right hemisphere)
- voluntary motor functioning
- attentional vigilance
- level of arousal
- motivation and self-drive or initiation of behavior

▶ **Parietal Lobes**
- sensory input from the body
- receptive language comprehension (usually left hemisphere)
- complex language processing (usually left hemisphere)
- reading, writing, and math processing (usually left hemisphere)
- visual-spatial functioning (usually right hemisphere)
- integration of sensory information (auditory, visual, and tactile)
- directed attention to visual, auditory, or tactile space

▶ **Temporal Lobes**
- auditory processing
- receptive language comprehension (usually left hemisphere)
- complex language processing (usually left hemisphere)
- prosody and intonation comprehension (usually right hemisphere)
- memory storage and retrieval
- emotional function
- instinctive drives involving fear, aggression, sexual behavior, hunger, etc.

▶ **Occipital Lobes**
- light perception
- perception or experience of seeing
- visual processing from simple to complex
- recognition of visual information (close to the temporal lobe)
- attention to visual space (close to the parietal lobe)

▶ **Allocortex/Limbic System**
- storage and retrieval of memories
- primitive emotional drives (e.g., aggression/defense, sexual behavior, predation/feeding)
- instinctive and species-specific behaviors (e.g., dominance-submission, approach-avoidance for mating and fighting)
- feelings of pleasure, rage, and fear

▶ **Thalamus**
- relays information between different parts of the brain
- processing and "gating" of information dependent on need (i.e., even though the sensory information from the skin always goes to the brain, often we do not notice this information; the thalamus helps you ignore the feeling of your watch strap, clothing, or a hat after a few seconds or minutes)

▶ **Hypothalamus**
- controls internal bodily states, such as emotion, hunger, thirst, body temperature, sexual/reproductive behavior, circadian rhythms, and the fight-or-flight response
- autonomic nervous system and hormonal system via pituitary function

▶ **Midbrain**
- contains nuclei and pathways that control movement, arousal, sleep, attention, muscle tone, pain and species-typical behaviors (e.g., mating, fighting); also includes areas that control visual and auditory orienting responses

▶ **Brain Stem**
- connects the brain with the spinal cord
- controls breathing, heartbeat, consciousness, and muscle tone
- movement of the eyes and mouth
- sensory information regarding temperature, pain, and hunger
- body temperature
- involuntary movement (e.g., sneezing, coughing, vomiting, swallowing)

▶ **Cerebellum**
- motor control involving coordination and timing
- muscle tone
- modulation of numerous cognitive processes, such as attention, memory, language, social awareness, and intellect

Often the brain is viewed from the top or sides. When brain imaging techniques such as MRI or CT scanners are used, the three-dimensional brain is drawn in two dimensions as a series of slices through the brain. The slices can be made using a sagittal cut, a coronal cut, or an axial cut. (See Notice to Our Readers on page 8.)

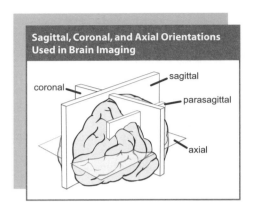

Sagittal, Coronal, and Axial Orientations Used in Brain Imaging

▶ Sagittal View

A *sagittal* cut is a vertical cut that is made from front to back down the length of the brain. A cut along the midsagittal plane divides the brain into the right and left hemispheres. Parasagittal slices cut down the length of the brain but not between the two hemispheres. Parasagittal slices show tissue within either the right or left hemisphere, depending on which one is being imaged.

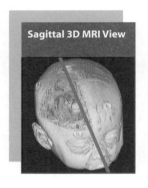
Sagittal 3D MRI View

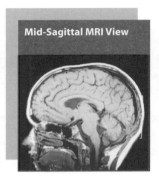
Mid-Sagittal MRI View

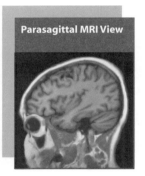
Parasagittal MRI View

▶ Coronal View

A *coronal* cut goes across the brain from one ear to the other. The cut divides the front from the back of the brain.

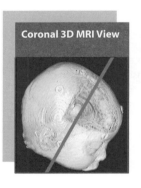
Coronal 3D MRI View

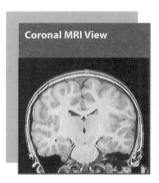
Coronal MRI View

▶ Axial View

An *axial* cut goes horizontally through the brain from front to back, separating a top portion of the brain from a bottom portion. The horizontal images or slices can be stacked on top of each other to make up the entire brain.

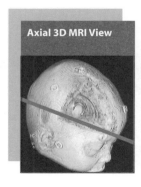
Axial 3D MRI View

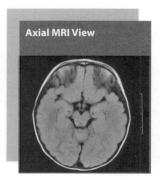
Axial MRI View

Chapter 2

Development of the Brain and Cognition

Brain development is influenced by both genetics and a child's interaction with other people and the environment. These interactions provide the child's evolving brain with a context to help guide future brain development. When a traumatic brain injury occurs during early development, it can change the course of neurodevelopment for a child.

It is difficult to assess cognitive and language functioning without having some idea of what is expected in normal development. A basic understanding of brain development, cognitive development, and the various effects of brain injury at different stages of development will help you understand the many limitations exhibited by children and adolescents following a TBI.

Note: We have provided a very general overview of brain development in this chapter because an in-depth explanation about brain growth is complex and beyond the scope of this book. We encourage you to research additional information on your own.

Brain Growth and Cognitive Development

The brain develops from the inside to the outside and from the back to the front as shown in the following chart.

Structure	Order of Development	Function
subcortical nuclei	first	made up of primitive brain cells that keep us alive
motor and sensory areas	second	allows us to interact with our environment
association areas of the parietal and frontal lobes	last	used to make sense of information and solve problems

Brain development involves five basic processes: proliferation, differentiation, arborization, myelination, and pruning.

1. Proliferation

Brain development begins with the formation of neurons (brain cells) and synapses (connections between brain cells) in the prenatal period. During this early phase of development, the brain produces more synapses than needed. This process is called *proliferation*.

The formation of synapses reaches it peak in the frontal cortex during early childhood. At this stage of brain development, infants and toddlers have approximately 50 percent more synapses than adults.

2. Differentiation

Early in the second trimester, at around four months of gestation, neurons move to specific areas of the brain where they are needed and become active members of functional systems. This is known as *differentiation*.

The process of differentiation accounts for the development of language and motor control functions during the first two years of life. At first, differentiation takes place in the structures that maintain life and in the primary sensory and motor areas. During late prenatal and postnatal development, differentiation takes place in the parietal lobes, the frontal lobes, and the cerebellum. These areas continue to differentiate well beyond birth and into early adulthood.

3. Arborization

Arborization is the process of dendritic branching. Dendrites are important for information processing. Dendrites form relatively slowly. They begin as individual bumps that jut out from a cell body. These bumps generate extensions that branch out to form tree-like structures. Small mushroom-like protrusions, called *spines*, begin to develop on the branches of some dendrites around the seventh month of gestation; however, most spines develop after a child is born in response to the child's interaction with the environment.

4. Myelination

Myelination is the process in which the communication fibers of the axons become covered with myelin. *Myelin* is the fatty substance, rich in protein and lipids, that surrounds and insulates nerve fibers. Myelination allows neurons to conduct signals more efficiently by increasing the speed of information transfer along axons to approximately 100 times that of non-myelinated cells.

Myelination is related to functional maturity and the development of cognitive skills. Although some areas of the brain myelinate before birth, the majority of myelination occurs in infancy and in early childhood. This accounts for the large increase in brain size and weight after a child is born. The brain areas responsible for decision making and judgment do not complete myelination until late adolescence to early adulthood.

> At birth, the brain is about one quarter of an adult-sized brain. By age two, the brain weighs approximately 2.8 lbs. (1300g), just less than an adult brain that weighs 3.0-3.3 lbs. (1400g to 1500g).

In general, myelin develops in the following pattern. Note that these are not absolute periods and some overlap in development of the different areas is expected.

■ Prenatal and Infant
- motor roots and sensory pathways
- spinal cord pathways

■ Postnatal Through Early Adulthood
- cortical to subcortical pathways (integrate information from areas of the cortex to areas below the cortex)
- cortical to cortical pathways (integrate information among areas of the cortex)
- callosal pathways (communicate between hemispheres)
- association areas of the frontal and parietal lobes (integrate motor and sensory functions)
- reticular activating system (maintains arousal and attentional vigilance)

5. Pruning

Pruning is the selective elimination of neurons and neural connections. Cells that are not needed die (*apoptosis*) and many synaptic connections disappear, leaving fewer, more efficient connections in place. Pruning begins in early childhood and continues until approximately 16 years of age. During adolescence, the brain becomes more efficient and needs fewer connections to do the work.

The brain develops at different rates, even at the cellular level. For example, neurons that communicate information long distances (*Golgi Type I*) mature before neurons that integrate information short distances (*Golgi Type II*). Development of Golgi Type I neurons corresponds with the early development of motor and sensory pathways. The slower development of Golgi Type II neurons corresponds to the later development of integrative areas that are used for problem solving.

Vulnerable periods, or *critical periods*, of brain development refer to times when the brain is going through rapid development related to one or more functions. Critical periods vary in length and are not exact. For example, the critical period for the processing of phonemes extends from approximately six months to nine months of age. At six months, a baby can produce and discriminate more than 90 known phonemes; however, by nine months the phonemes that the baby can discriminate have been pruned to only those sounds he has heard (approximately 38 for English).

Brain growth, especially the development of cognitive abilities, coordinates with a child's functional development. Increases in brain weight coincide with irregular growth periods in physical development called *growth spurts*. During these times, there is no real increase in the number of brain cells; therefore, the weight increase is most likely due to the branching and growth of the dendrites in addition to the formation of myelination around the axons. Development of cognitive skills tends to occur with these changes, with the increased brain weight corresponding to rapid advances in cognitive ability, or *cognitive growth spurts*.

Age of Growth Spurt	% Increase in Brain Weight	General Cognitive Development
3 to 10 months	30%	infantile reflexes
2 to 4 years	5 – 10%	symbolic language/visual-motor integration
6 to 8 years	5 – 10%	beginning of abstract reasoning
10 to 12 years	5 – 10%	abstract conceptualization of information
14 to 16+ years	5 – 10%	conceptual and integrated thinking

Symbolic language develops between the ages of two and four years. During these early years, children think by using associations, such as *A cow says, "moo"* or *A cow lives on a farm.*

Between six to eight years, children begin to think abstractly and their responses are more conceptual. They make statements, such as *A cow is an animal that gives milk.*

By 10 to 12 years of age, their thinking is primarily abstract. Responses are more complex. For example, if you ask, "What is a firefighter?" the child may respond, "Someone who rescues people and puts out fires," rather than, "Someone who helps people, wears a hat, and rides in a big red truck."

Adolescents have fully developed conceptual thinking skills and can process abstract problems, such as those presented in algebra (e.g., $2x + 5 = 35$ $x =$ __).

Studies using functional imaging techniques, such as positron emission tomography (PET) scans, show that metabolic activity varies in different regions of the brain at different ages of development.

- In newborns, most activity happens in the sensory-motor cortex and the brain stem, relating to the basic sensory-motor and arousal functions of the baby.

- At two to three months, metabolic activity is prominent in the sensory-parietal cortices as the baby begins to process information from the environment.

- Between six months and one year, metabolic activity is marked in the frontal cortex, helping the child interact with the environment and other people.

Eventually, as the child develops, more areas of the brain become involved as a result of improved integration of the many brain regions.

Piaget's Stages of Cognitive Development

Most courses on child development rely heavily on Piaget's stages of cognitive development. Because Piaget's terminology has become standard for the field of child development, it will be helpful for you to review his stages and note how brain growth spurts relate to his findings.

Age Range	Developmental Stage	General Characteristics of the Stage
0 to 2 years	Sensorimotor	• Cognitive system limited to sensory/motor functioning
2 to 6 years	Preoperational	• Capable of mental representation but not organized thinking
7 to 11 years	Concrete operational	• Intelligence is logical and symbolic
12 to Adult	Formal operational	• Capable of formulating hypotheses and testing them against reality

Normal Developmental Milestones

A developmental milestones chart for cognitive development, gross-motor development, fine-motor development, self-help skills, social development, expressive language development, and receptive language development can be found in Appendix 2A, page 38. Please note that the ages of development are approximate.

Common Labels Used to Describe Approximate Age Ranges

It is helpful to use a relatively standardized nomenclature to refer to children of different ages and developmental stages. Here is a list of common labels used for the different age ranges of children. All ages are approximations.

Terminology Relating to a Child's Age:
- Prenatal—Conception to approximately 280 days (approximately 40 weeks)
- Neonate—Birth to first postnatal month
- Infant—1 month to 12 months
- Toddler—1 year to 2 years-11 months
- Early Childhood (Preschooler)—3 years to 5 years-11 months
- Later Childhood (School-Age)—6 years to 12 years
- Preadolescence/Adolescence—10 to18 years
- Puberty (Girls)—approximately 13 years
- Puberty (Boys)—approximately 15 years

How Does a Brain Injury Affect Normal Brain Development?

The effects of injury to a developing brain are complex and difficult to understand without taking into account developmental factors. Damage to the brain can have different effects depending on the child's age and stage of development. Therefore, developmental changes taking place during the time of a child's injury should be considered when assessing functioning. Changes in brain organization from ongoing development should also be taken into account when predicting future difficulties related to any disruption of the developmental processes.

Early in development, the brain is immature and the cells have not completed their differentiation and structural organization. A focal, or localized, injury at this stage can result in generalized deficits and slowed cognitive development. If there is injury to an area of the brain necessary for a skill or learning that develops later in childhood, impairments related to that skill may not become evident until many years later.

As a general rule, the younger the child, the more likely damage from a TBI will cause diffuse deficits. Because the brain of an infant is not yet specialized, a brain injury during infancy can cause diffuse disruption of brain and cognitive functioning. It can also disrupt normal development, which in turn can disrupt a variety of functions. In an older child, it is more likely that the damage will cause deficits involving specific abilities. A similar injury in an older person may cause more focal, or localized neurological problems, and cognitive deficits, such as an aphasia.

For example, an infant with a brain injury may quickly recover the ability to use single-word utterances, such as *juice* or *up*, but may fail to develop normal language. This impairment may only become apparent in later childhood when verbal reasoning and the use of complex, language-based information is required for learning. The child may then be thought of as having a language-based learning disability.

A child who becomes brain injured at a young age or during critical periods of brain development often may have a different rate of cognitive development later in life. The child ages at the same rate as his peers but the rate of development is slower. Because a child with a brain injury often lags behind his peers in development, the gap widens between his achievement levels and those of other students in school. A child's measured IQ score may decline as the child gets older because he is learning at a rate slower than his peers. If a TBI occurs in a child during a critical period, deficits may be more pronounced, with specific loss of skills that were undergoing rapid development.

A focal injury during later childhood or adolescence causes deficits that usually involve only those skills related to the specific area(s) of brain damage. Specific deficits show up because there is damage to pre-existing functions that were relatively mature. The child often retains old learning and skills that can help him compensate for his new deficits. This intact, old learning can give others the impression that the child has recovered fully from his injury. Unfortunately, ongoing deficits relating to new learning or executive functioning may persist indefinitely.

A diffuse, or widespread injury typically results in a global disruption of functional skills regardless of the age of the child at the time of injury. Cognitive deficits in young children after a diffuse injury may not become apparent until many years later when they are not able to meet age-appropriate expectancies for increasingly difficult skills. For example, a child may quickly recover the ability to communicate verbally or understand basic tables, but fail to develop the ability to conceptualize linguistic information abstractly or do higher-level visual reasoning involving geometry.

Research on Brain Development

Some of the earliest research concerning the effects of brain injury on the developing brain was conducted by researchers Margaret Kennard, Donald Hebb, and John Dobbing. Their findings help explain why many children who have early brain injuries appear to recover soon after an injury but have long-standing difficulties later in childhood. (See Appendix 2B, page 39, for more detailed information on their research and theories.)

▶ Cognitive Development

- explores environment via senses .... birth-6 months
- uses simple actions to explore .... 5-9 months
- finds objects that are hidden .... 7-9 months
- imitates a variety of simple actions ...... 9-13 months
- uses objects purposefully .... 12-18 months
- uses trial-and-error to solve problems ... 12-18 months
- uses imaginative play .... 18-24 months
- completes a simple puzzle .... 24-36 months
- imitates multi-step routines .... 24-36 months
- matches pictures and objects .... 24-36 months
- knows basic quantity and size concepts 3.0-4.0 years
- categorizes objects/pictures .... 4.0-5.0 years
- completes simple matrices .... 4.0-5.0 years
- identifies missing parts of objects ...... 4.2-5.6 years
- makes object associations .... 4.6-5.6 years
- sequences story pictures .... 4.6-5.6 years

▶ Gross-Motor Development

- sits independently .... 5-9 months
- crawls on hands and knees .... 9-12 months
- pulls to stand .... 9-12 months
- walks .... 11-14 months
- runs .... 14-20 months
- kicks ball .... 17-22 months
- stands on one foot .... 30-36 months
- pedals tricycle .... 3.0-3.6 years
- hops on one foot .... 3.6-4.0 years
- demonstrates heel-toe walking .... 4.0-5.6 years

▶ Fine-Motor Development

- demonstrates thumb-finger
  pincer grasp .... 9-12 months
- scribbles with crayons .... 12-18 months
- stacks two or more blocks .... 12-18 months
- turns pages of a book .... 18-24 months
- makes circles with a crayon .... 24-30 months
- imitates a vertical line .... 30-36 months
- copies a circle .... 3.0-3.6 years
- copies a square .... 4.0-5.0 years
- draws a person .... 4.0-5.0 years

▶ Self-Help Skills

- drinks from cup .... 9-18 months
- spoon feeds .... 12-18 months
- removes clothing .... 12-20 months
- dresses self with help .... 30-36 months
- washes and dries hands .... 30-36 months
- dresses without help .... 3.0-4.0 years
- toileting .... by 5.0 years

▶ Social Development

- plays social games .... 9-12 months
- sometimes says "No" .... 18-24 months
- responds to correction .... 18-24 months
- plays pretend games .... 30-36 months
- plays cooperatively .... 3.6-4.0 years
- plays games with rules .... 4.6-5.0 years

▶ Expressive Language Development

- *Mama/Dada* specifically .... 8-10 months
- babbles with intonation .... 10-18 months
- uses one to two words .... 11-13 months
- uses mature jargoning .... 16-24 months
- puts two words together .... 18-26 months
- has a 50-word vocabulary .... 18-24 months
- uses pronouns .... 2.6-3.6 years
- states first name .... 2.6-3.6 years
- combines sentences .... 3.0-4.0 years
- names four colors .... 3.0-4.0 years
- speaks clearly .... 3.6-4.6 years
- asks questions for information .... 3.8-4.2 years
- participates in conversation .... 4.6-5.0 years

▶ Receptive Language Development

- responds to "No" .... 9-12 months
- points to three body parts .... 13-18 months
- follows one-part command .... 16-20 months
- follows two-part commands .... 20-30 months
- understands pronouns .... 24-30 months
- understands concept of "one" .... 24-30 months
- understands basic prepositions .... 30-38 months
- identifies four colors .... 3.6-4.0 years
- understands action words .... 3.6-4.6 years
- counts five or more objects .... 3.6-4.6 years
- begins reading single letters .... 4.6-5.0 years

▶ **Margaret Kennard** (late 1930s and early 1940s)

Kennard evaluated the effects of brain injuries in young monkeys. She noticed that injuries in infant monkeys did not cause the same permanent motor impairment as seen in adult monkeys with similar injuries.

Kennard's work resulted in the development of the *Kennard Principal*, a theory regarding the sparing and recovery of function following brain injury in infants. According to Kennard, the optimal time to sustain a cortical lesion, in regard to recovery of motor impairment, is early in development. She believed that early injuries were less disabling than those received later in life.

A great deal of research following this early work supported Kennard's conclusions. Thus, the Kennard Principal gained widespread acceptance even though the studies were limited to animals and primarily to the motor system. Consequently, caution should be used when relating Kennard's results to children who are developing.

▶ **Donald Hebb** (1940s)

Hebb conducted studies involving childhood development and brain injury. He noticed that children who had brain injuries in infancy and early childhood had a higher risk of poor outcomes later in life. Hebb's work suggested that early injuries can disrupt development with the effects of the injury becoming apparent many years later.

▶ **John Dobbing** (1960s and 1970s)

Dobbing used primates to study theories, such as those developed by Hebb. Dobbing found that many of the primates that were brain injured early in life showed impairments in functioning later in life. His research indicated that the course of development had been interrupted by the early injury. Dobbing developed a second theory regarding age and TBI, known as the *Dobbing Hypothesis*. The Dobbing Hypothesis suggests that brain damage has its greatest influence on development when it takes place during vulnerable developmental periods.

Chapter 3

Traumatic Brain Injury

Traumatic brain injury is "an acquired injury to the brain caused by external physical force, resulting in total or partial functional disability or psychosocial impairment, or both, that adversely affects a child's educational performance. The term applies to open or closed head injuries resulting in impairments in one or more areas, such as cognition; language; memory; attention; reasoning; abstract thinking; judgment; problem solving; sensory, perceptual and motor abilities; psychosocial behavior; physical functions; information processing; and speech. The term does not apply to brain injuries that are congenital or degenerative, or to brain injuries induced by birth trauma."

The Individuals with Disabilities Education Act (IDEA), Public Law 101-476,
Amended December 3, 2004: Public Law 108-446, Code of Federal Regulations (CFR) for Title 34

Facts Regarding TBI in Children and Adolescents

- Each year, approximately 16 million children are treated in emergency departments and 600,000 children are hospitalized due to TBI-related injuries.

- For children between the ages of 1 to 19 years, unintentional injuries are the number one cause of death (17/100,000).

- Data from multiple trauma centers shows that approximately 75%-97% of pediatric trauma deaths result from TBI.

- The most common cause of pediatric TBI is motor vehicle collisions (i.e., acceleration-deceleration injuries that occur when the head accelerates and then suddenly stops), followed by falls, recreational activities, and assault.

- TBI is the number one cause of disability in children and young adults.

- Males are about 1.5 times as likely as females to sustain a TBI.

- The two age groups at highest risk for TBI are 0- to 4-year-olds and 15- to 19-year-olds.

General Information Regarding Brain Injury

A *traumatic brain injury* (TBI) is an injury to the brain that is caused by the head striking against or being struck by an object, by violent shaking, or by other methods that inflict trauma, such as a gunshot wound. The term *TBI* is not used for a person who is born with a brain injury, who incurs a brain injury caused by birth trauma or infection, or who has problems with brain development.

There is no such thing as a typical brain injury. TBIs affect different parts of the brain, vary in severity from mild (i.e., a brief change in mental status or loss of consciousness) to severe (i.e., an extended period of coma), and result in different symptoms for each child. A TBI can change how a child acts, moves, feels, and/or processes information.

The following chart outlines the common complaints expressed by children and adolescents with TBI and the cognitive, physical, and emotional difficulties they may experience one or more years post injury.

Common Complaints

- difficulty with memory and problem-solving skills
- problems managing stress and emotional upsets, such as controlling one's temper
- slowed speed of thinking and more time needed to take tests and do tasks
- difficulty learning in school
- poor ability to improve skills necessary for academic or vocational advancement

Cognitive Difficulties	Physical Difficulties	Emotional Difficulties
• arousal and alertness • orientation to person, place, time, and situation • attention and concentration • thinking and problem solving • verbal and nonverbal reasoning ability • intelligence • abstraction and concept formation • language and communicative functioning (receptive and expressive) • visual perception • memory and learning • judgment and decision making • processing speed • executive functioning • rigidity of thought and perseveration (i.e., difficulty thinking "outside the box") • auditory and visual processing • academic skills	• regulation of automatic bodily functions (e.g., temperature) • motor strength • motor coordination • sequencing of motor skills • balance and the ability to walk • energy level or endurance • tightness of muscles • inability to stop muscle movements (i.e., prevent tremors) • sensitivity to touch • sexual dysfunction • eye function • seizures • speech production • eating and swallowing	• emotional lability • agitation and irritability • low frustration tolerance • anger outbursts • flat affect • depression

A summary of symptoms and disorders relating to various areas of the brain is provided in Appendix 3A, pages 64-65.

Often, the parts of the brain that are damaged are more critical than the size of the brain injury. For example, a microscopic injury in a specific area of the brain may cause a prolonged vegetative state while a large, diffuse (widespread) injury may only result in mild deficits.

Limitations following a brain injury can involve many aspects of functioning depending on the severity of the injury and the specific areas of the brain that are involved. Brain injuries can lead to impairments involving cognitive functioning, motor functioning, sensory functioning, language skills, behavior, and/or emotion. Most of the time, however, an injury will result in reduced efficiency when performing normal functions rather than a loss of functioning altogether. In other words, the ability is neither present nor absent; rather there is a change in the child's ability to function.

Unique Aspects of TBI

TBIs are qualitatively different from injuries to other parts of the body. A broken arm often heals completely, its symptoms are consistent across environments, and the rate of recovery is generally the same across patients. In contrast, difficulties experienced by patients with TBI vary dramatically and may be inconsistent across environments. Common features of TBI include:

- The condition is chronic and complete recovery is rare.

- Life for the patient is changed forever.

- Cognitive deficits may not be obvious to others after recovery from physical injuries. The patient may walk, talk, and look normal, but he may not think normally.

- Deficits from the injury may not become apparent until many years after the injury.

- Symptoms are inconsistent due to intact old learning and the impaired ability to learn new information.

- Often there is loss of some cognitive functions.

- Damage to one brain system may impact functioning in other brain areas.

- Attention and executive-functioning deficits can make performance fluctuate from one occasion to another (e.g., moment to moment, day to day, week to week).

- The patient may be able to do difficult tasks but not easier ones (e.g., a child may be able to do difficult math problems but may not be able to name common objects).

- Changes in the rate of recovery make planning for accommodations difficult.

- It is difficult to tell which problems are related to the brain injury and which are normal for the child's age.

Causes of Brain Damage Resulting from TBI

The physical force of a TBI can cause the following traumas within the brain.

- direct physical impact or bouncing of the brain inside the skull (e.g., coup/contrecoup)

- penetration and tearing of tissue (e.g., bullet, skull fragments)

- shear injury from diffuse physical forces acting on the brain

- bleeding caused by tearing of blood vessels

- increased intracranial pressure from acute blood vessel dilation

- increased intracranial pressure hours to days later due to *edema* (increased fluid/swelling)

- reduced blood flow and cell loss due to lack of oxygen

- seizures that increase the metabolic rate of the brain by a factor of 10; *hypoxia* (oxygen deficiency) sets in when the blood flow cannot keep up with the increased metabolic rate

- herniation of the brain, which occurs when brain tissue is pushed across a membrane (e.g., dura)

- hypoxic injury due to respiratory arrest as a result of brain stem damage or increased intracranial pressure

> Hypoxic injuries resulting from seizures or TBI-related respiratory arrest generally have a worse prognosis than a purely traumatic injury without hypoxia. Hypoxic injuries can affect the entire brain and involve all of the brain cells.

Note: See page 46 for more information on coup and contrecoup injuries.
    See pages 47-48 for more information on penetrating injuries.
    See page 50 for more information on shear injury.

Trauma to the brain often results in microscopic damage to the cells and their connections.

Cellular Damage

Severely damaged neurons in the area of a brain injury eventually die. The non-injured cells adapt and grow new connections to overcome the disruption of functions that results from these dying cells. If only a few cells die in an area, the other cells in that area can make new connections and take over the work; however, when many cells die, it is harder for the brain to compensate for the damage. In addition, most areas of the brain have specialized functions and are comprised of specialized types of cells. The cells in each area are different or are organized differently, so they cannot take over functions for other damaged areas.

Damage to the Communication Pathways (Axons)

The brain is like a large ball of fibers that interconnect and communicate with each other, making it a fully integrated system. When there is an injury, damage in one area of the brain will often cause disruption to functions in areas without damage. A particular function may be disrupted by damage to the area of the brain that controls that function, by damage to the other areas it communicates with, or by damage to the communication pathways that connect the two areas.

Damage to the communication pathways of the brain can be as disruptive to brain function as damage to specific areas of the brain. Difficulties caused by poor communication between brain areas often become evident when processing demands increase above a basic level. A child with intact receptive and expressive language functioning may have little difficulty with basic communication. The child's deficits may not become apparent until he is asked to perform tasks involving verbal abstraction, such as describing how two words are similar. Loss of communication pathways in the brain may make it difficult for the child to integrate information that is required to make abstract associations between two things.

When communication pathways are damaged, information cannot move from one area to another quickly and processing speed slows down. It is similar to driving from one side of a major metropolitan city to another, using side streets instead of freeways. When communication pathways are damaged, it is as if the "freeways" of the brain are under construction. The information transmission is forced to use less efficient pathways that require more energy and more time.

The reduced communication efficiency accounts for some of the slower information processing seen after a brain injury. The extra effort it takes to do a task is also why children with brain injuries have difficulty multitasking or rapidly switching between tasks. So much energy and so many resources are required for one task that the child is unable to do more than one thing at a time, or efficiently switch between multiple tasks. Energy resources are quickly used up, and fatigue can build rapidly.

Note: See page 15 for a table of the main communication pathways.

> Microscopic damage may not be visible on a brain scan. This does not mean that the damage did not take place; it only means that the scan is not sensitive enough to visualize microscopic details. Sometimes, microscopic damage across the entire brain can be devastating even though the child has normal brain scans.

Effects of Trauma on the Brain

In general, brain injuries of comparable type and severity result in a similar profile of deficits; however, there are always exceptions. Because no two children have exactly the same brain anatomy (organizational structure), two injuries of the same severity may have very different outcomes (i.e., two children may have damage to the same area of the brain but show different symptoms).

Most of the time, TBI results in disruption of one or more of the following functions.

- motor execution
- sensation
- language
- vision
- memory
- thinking
- bodily functions (e.g., arousal from coma, blood pressure, breathing)

The location of the TBI is a factor in determining which functional deficits may be present. For example, injuries to the frontal and medial temporal lobes generally result in deficits involving executive functioning and memory. Left hemisphere injuries normally disrupt language functioning while right hemisphere injuries commonly result in the disruption of visual-spatial functions. An injury to the back of the brain will usually disrupt visual processing.

Brain damage can be localized (*focal*) to a specific brain region and/or diffuse, with the injury affecting multiple brain areas. For example, a closed head injury may have some focal features (e.g., motor paralysis of the arm) as well as some diffuse symptoms, such as poor executive functioning. Similarly, a penetrating injury caused by a high-speed projectile, such as a bullet, may result in focal injury to the brain within the path of the bullet and diffuse injury as a result of the shock wave produced by the bullet traveling through the soft brain tissue. Although most TBIs can have a variety of features, clinically, it is helpful to think of the damage and symptoms as being in one of the quadrants depicted to the right.

	Focal	**Diffuse**
Closed Head	A	B
Penetrating	C	D

A = closed head injury with focal damage
B = closed head injury with diffuse damage
C = penetrating injury with focal damage
D = penetrating injury with diffuse damage

Closed Head Injury

A *closed head injury* can be defined as a trauma to the brain without penetration of the skull. Closed head injuries can result from:

- the head striking against an object
- the head being hit by an object
- the head moving rapidly enough so that brain tissue becomes twisted due to rotational forces

Secondary damage can occur when the brain hits the hard and sometimes sharp, bony structures on the inner surface of the skull. Because of irregularities inside the skull, some areas of the brain are more likely to be injured than others. Areas prone to additional damage include the underside of the frontal lobes just above the eye orbits and the front portion of the temporal lobes because they are surrounded by bony protrusions.

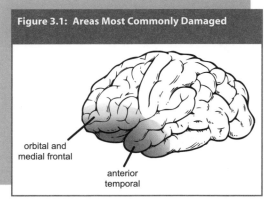

Figure 3.1: Areas Most Commonly Damaged

orbital and medial frontal

anterior temporal

The movement of the brain may cause tearing or *shearing* as the brain tissues twist out of shape. These tissues can also be crushed against bone causing *contusions* (bruises) in the brain. Typically there is less injury to the brain in the areas where the inside of the skull is smooth.

Because brain tissue is soft, physical forces acting on the brain can damage more than one area. For example, during a car accident, the driver may hit the left side of his head on the car door, causing an injury to his skull and brain on the left side (*coup* injury). Damage may also occur on the side opposite the impact (*contrecoup* injury) when, after the driver hits the left side of his head, his brain moves rapidly and bounces to the other side of his skull, causing bruising on the right side of his brain.

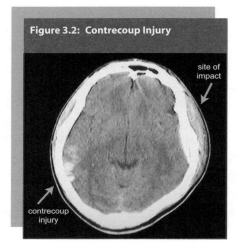

Figure 3.2: Contrecoup Injury

site of impact

contrecoup injury

In a closed head injury, the chances for infection are minimal because there is no opening to the brain; however, these types of injuries are likely to result in loss of consciousness.

Case Example 1 *Juan*

Juan was 14 years old when he was hit by a truck moving at a high rate of speed. Juan had multiple physical injuries and a severe closed head brain injury. He was in a coma for many weeks.

Once he was medically stable and his family was trained to care for him, Juan was discharged from the hospital. At the time of his discharge, Juan was only able to open his eyes and squeeze Dr. Lebby's hand in response to verbal requests. Juan had no other cognitive abilities. He required medications to wake up during the day and injections of Botox to relax the spasticity in his muscles. Almost three months later, he came back to our clinic for a follow-up assessment. At that time he was able to say a few words, including his name and age. He could also tell us that he was at the hospital and he was hungry.

Juan, continued

Because Juan was able to follow a few simple directions and say a few words, he was readmitted to the hospital for inpatient rehabilitation. After several weeks of intensive rehabilitation, he was able to talk about simple topics and follow a sequence of directions. He also made significant improvements in his motor functioning (e.g., learning to walk using a walker); however, his memory was very poor and he was unable to function without external guidance and structure.

Unfortunately, Juan then suffered an onset of seizures that caused the loss of many of the gains he had made. Following medical stabilization, he began to improve again. When Juan left the rehabilitation unit approximately six weeks later, he was able to walk and give his name, his age, and his location, but little else. His memory remained impaired and he did not remember what he did from day to day.

Juan's story is all too common. Many children are injured in similar ways each year. Other children and adolescents may sustain head injuries that are less severe than Juan's, but are just as disabling. In general, a brain injury that is severe enough to result in hospitalization will affect the child's future functioning in some way. Even mild injuries can result in subtle changes to a child's motor, cognitive, and/or emotional functioning.

Penetrating Injury

In a *penetrating injury*, something breaks into the skull. This type of injury can cause damage all along the path of the penetrating object as it tears nerve fibers, blood vessels, and other brain tissues.

The child may or may not lose consciousness from a penetrating injury. If he does not lose consciousness, do not assume that his injury is minor. Significant brain damage and cognitive deficits may occur without a loss of consciousness.

Neurologic signs are often related only to the functions of the area damaged (e.g., specific motor impairment, language impairment, etc.). Recovery is often rapid, although children will frequently have long-term deficits related to the areas of injury. The deficits can range from very mild with no notable impairments, to a loss of critical functions required for life.

As the foreign object tears through the brain tissue, it may or may not cause additional injury radiating from its path. For example, slow-moving projectiles (e.g., bone being pushed into the brain from a skull fracture, objects penetrating the brain from a car accident, and pellets or BBs piercing the brain from a shooting accident) generally only cause damage close to the channel created by the object.

On the other hand, faster-moving objects, such as a high velocity bullet, can cause a shock wave that travels away from the trajectory of the bullet. The shock wave results in more diffuse axonal injury or shear injury and can even liquefy the substance of the brain due to heat dispersion, severely damaging cellular structures and resulting in the formation of a large cavity within the brain. Bullet fragments can also damage multiple areas of the brain as they tear through tissue. Secondary complications from penetration injuries include blood loss and the risk of infection.

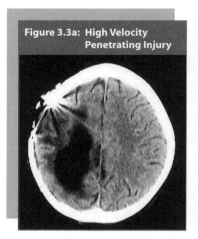

Figure 3.3a: High Velocity Penetrating Injury

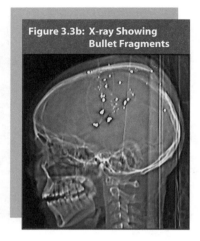

Figure 3.3b: X-ray Showing Bullet Fragments

Case Example 2 *Sharon*

Sharon, a three-year-old, was accidentally shot in the head with a pellet gun. Even though the pellet had approximately the same circumference as the bullet that caused the damage depicted in Figure 3.3a, Sharon sustained less damage because the pellet was moving much slower. (See Figure 3.4.) The pellet penetrated her skull, traveled from her right frontal lobe through her brain tissue, and ultimately came to rest in the left side of her cerebellum. This resulted in a low-velocity, penetrating brain injury because the pellet had slowed substantially by the time it penetrated her skull.

Interestingly, when we entered Sharon's hospital room only a few hours after her injury, we were pleasantly surprised to see her sitting in bed playing with her parents. She was immediately communicative and was able to tell us her name, who her parents were, and what she was playing. Her deficits were very specific to the areas of the brain that were damaged by the path of the pellet.

Sharon's TBI resulted in specific deficits involving motor functioning for her left side, but she had no other apparent cognitive or physical limitations. Sharon left the hospital a few weeks later with a mild left hemiparesis (partial paralysis) and some hormonal difficulties due to damage to her pituitary gland and pituitary stalk. She has since demonstrated normal cognitive development because the pellet did not damage the areas of her brain used for cognition.

Figure 3.4: Low Velocity Penetrating Injury

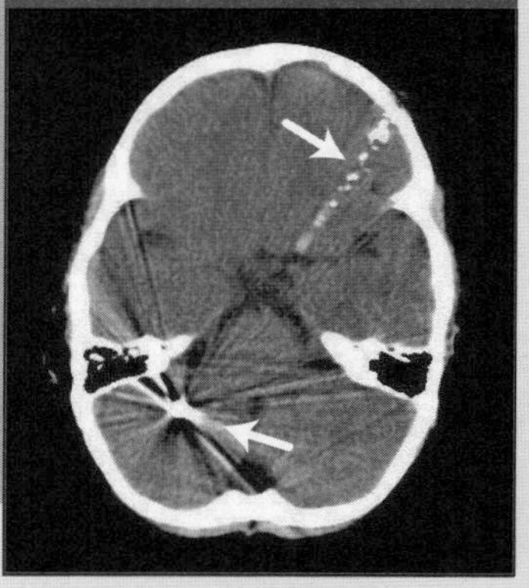

Pellet path is visible on scan; bone and blood show up in lighter shade than brain tissue. Starburst at back of brain represents CT artifact from metal pellet. Center of starburst shows where pellet came to rest.

Focal Damage

Damage involving a small, localized area of the brain is called a *focal injury*. Deficits from focal damage depend on the site and severity of the injury. These injuries involve limited brain sites and include:

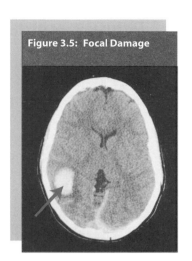

Figure 3.5: Focal Damage

- *contusions* (bruises of the brain)
- *hematomas* (bleeds in the brain)
- physical destruction of tissue from a penetrating object

It is uncommon for a TBI to result only in focal damage because the extreme physical forces involved with most TBIs cause diffuse damage. Some injuries, however, are identified as being more focal in nature due to the symptoms that are most evident. Even if symptoms are restricted to one or two cognitive processes, microscopic damage to other areas of the brain is almost always present.

Diffuse Damage

Damage involving multiple areas of the brain is called a *diffuse injury*. Diffuse injuries often result in the disruption of many brain processes, diminishing the child's ability to perform a variety of cognitive tasks. Diffuse injuries include:

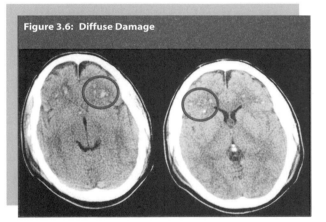

Figure 3.6: Diffuse Damage

Two different brain scans showing diffuse injury to the frontal lobes. The light spots show where the tearing of brain tissue was most severe (highlighted circles).

- *diffuse axonal injury* (ripping or tearing of nerve cells)
- brain swelling (increased fluid in the skull)

A child with a diffuse brain injury may have little or no evidence of physical trauma (e.g., a skull fracture). That is because diffuse injuries involve the internal structures of the brain. The lack of evidence of physical trauma does not relate to the severity of the injury; severe and even fatal brain injuries can occur without external evidence of trauma.

Mild diffuse injuries can be more disabling than a severe focal injury to a part of the brain that is not required for critical functions. For example, a diffuse injury may result in impaired executive functioning, which is very disruptive to a child's performance in school. A severe focal injury to a small region of the occipital lobe may only result in a visual loss that is extremely mild and does not limit the child in any way.

49

Diffuse Axonal Injury (Shear Injury)

For many TBIs, the tearing of tissue is responsible for the majority of symptoms. This type of tearing is known as *shear injury*, *diffuse axonal injury (DAI)*, *axonal shear injury*, or *diffuse shear injury*.

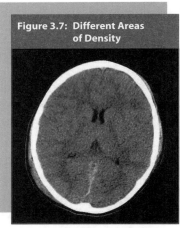

Figure 3.7: Different Areas of Density

Rotational or rapid acceleration-deceleration forces acting on the brain increase the chances of diffuse shear injuries. Areas of the brain have different densities of cells or tissue. For example, white matter, which is composed mostly of fatty myelin, has a different density than grey matter, which is made up of cell bodies. When a physical force acts on tissues with different densities, the tissues tend to move at different rates and/or in different directions. Similarly, when the brain is shaken or struck on something hard, the different parts of the brain move next to each other or slide back and forth at different speeds, causing the connections (axons) between the parts to tear or pull apart.

CT scans work like X-rays. Denser tissue absorbs the most X-rays and appears white on the CT image. Less dense tissue absorbs fewer X-rays and looks darker.

Loss of Consciousness and Coma

Injury to some parts of the brain often results in a loss of consciousness. This can range from a very brief period of poor awareness to a prolonged period of *unconsciousness* or *vegetative state*, called a *coma*. Coma is a sleep-like state in which the child does not speak, follow directions, or show purposeful and functional use of the limbs. Initially, most children in a coma do not open their eyes. With time, however, a child may develop eye opening and even sleep-wake cycles.

The primary cause for loss of consciousness is bilateral diffuse axonal injury (shear injury). It can also be caused by injury to the brain stem structures that regulate arousal. Although some penetrating injuries do not initially cause unconsciousness, secondary injury to the brain from swelling or *hemorrhage* (bleeding) can cause a delayed loss of consciousness. Even without loss of consciousness, penetrating injuries can result in severe brain damage and severe cognitive deficits.

When injury involves the brain stem, the loss of consciousness can last for many days or weeks. This is because fibers running through the brain stem give us our ability to waken and stay aroused during the day. Most children wake up slowly from a coma, with gradual improvements in arousal, cognitive skills, and motor functions. Over the few weeks that it takes most children to wake from a coma, memory for new learning is disrupted and the child has limited or no awareness of what goes on.

Some injuries put strain on the brain stem fibers, rather than permanently damaging them. Coma caused by strain to the brain stem fibers often resolves quickly with the child demonstrating rapid return of normal arousal and cognitive skills. This type of injury is called a *light switch injury* because the child wakes up from the coma suddenly, as if someone turned on a light switch.

The length of time someone remains unconscious has been related to the severity of the injury. In general, the longer someone is in a coma, the worse the brain injury and the outcome. Children who wake up from an extended coma require medical and therapeutic intervention for many weeks. Most never regain independent functioning and usually remain disabled for the rest of their lives. With a short period of coma, outcomes can vary a great deal, making it more difficult to predict how a child will function.

It is important to note whether the coma was caused by the accident or if it was medically induced. Sometimes a patient is prescribed medications to put him into a comatose state. A medication-induced coma is used to prevent movement if there is a spinal cord injury and to control medical conditions, such as increased intracranial pressure. If the coma is medically-induced, the relationship between the length of the coma and the severity and extent of the brain injury is less reliable.

Descriptions of the various states of coma are often based on the child's level of awareness (which is cortically mediated) and his level of arousal (which is a brain stem mediated function). Awareness involves a child's ability to process, integrate, and make sense of internally generated information and external environmental stimuli. A child demonstrates awareness when he exhibits goal-directed or purposeful behaviors and/or appropriate, specific responses to stimulation that he replicates in a consistent manner. Arousal, on the other hand, is a very primitive brain stem reflex that is often preserved in children with severe brain injuries. A child may have good arousal because of preserved brain stem functioning, but no awareness because there is severe damage to his cortex.

- *Consciousness* is a state in which the child has both intact arousal and awareness.

- Children in a *minimally-conscious state* generally have intact arousal mechanisms with inconsistent or disrupted awareness. They may also have appropriate sleep-wake cycles. Patients may respond to the environment and exhibit cognitively-mediated behavior consistently enough for clinicians to distinguish it from unconscious, reflexive responses.

- Children in a *persistent vegetative state* generally have intact arousal mechanisms and sometimes appropriate sleep-wake cycles but deficient awareness (they do not exhibit purposeful behaviors or consistent responses to stimulation).

- Children in a deep *coma* can be thought of as having deficient functioning involving both their arousal mechanism and their awareness.

Levels of Traumatic Brain Injury

Traumatic brain injuries can range from very mild, in which there is only one to two minutes of cognitive disruption, to severe, in which there is profound permanent disruption of brain functioning. In general, injuries of increasing severity affect deeper and deeper structures in the brain. The severity and symptoms of brain injury are often correlated with the level of brain injury, as follows:

- **Mild** TBIs cause mostly transient disruption of cortical functioning.

- **Moderate** TBIs cause damage to the cortex and the deeper structures of the diencephalon and mesencephalon.

- **Severe** TBIs often cause damage to all levels of the brain from the cortex to the diencephalon, midbrain, and brain stem.

Mild Traumatic Brain Injury

A mild traumatic brain injury may or may not have a brief loss of consciousness. If there is no loss of consciousness, there will be some alteration of mental status, such as a period of confusion and/or disorientation.

A TBI is generally considered mild if the child exhibits one or more of the following features.

- loss of consciousness no longer than 20 to 30 minutes

- Glasgow Coma Scale (GCS) score greater than 12
  The Glasgow Coma Scale is a tool used to measure acute brain injury. It has scores ranging from 3 (no functioning) to 15 (normal functioning). A copy of this scale is provided on the CD-ROM.

- no evidence of physical brain injury on neuroimaging

- less than an hour of post-traumatic amnesia (inability to store and retrieve new information)

- less than two days of hospitalization relating to the brain injury (not physical injuries)

Because loss of consciousness may only last a few minutes, you should be cautious when using the GCS score with mild TBIs. If you measure the GCS approximately 30 minutes or more after an injury, it may indicate a normal score of 15 even though there was an initial loss of consciousness. We also recommend that you use caution when reviewing brain imaging studies. Mild TBIs do not show up on brain scans, so the adage of *absence of evidence is not evidence of absence* should be considered when assessing such data.

Changes in a child's mental status involving behavioral and cognitive functioning are better indicators of a mild traumatic brain injury than brain scans. You can also use evidence from witnesses at the scene or information from the first responders, suggesting a brief loss of consciousness or confusion, to confirm a mild TBI. Difficulty with memory for new information, slowed mental processing speed, and reduced cognitive efficiency can also suggest that the child suffered a mild TBI.

Symptoms of mild TBI most often resolve in a day or two but can persist for several weeks. In a small minority of cases, a mild TBI can result in deterioration of neurological functioning as a result of medical complications, such as a slow bleed or slow increase in intracranial pressure which may become life-threatening.

Concussion

The terms *concussion* and *mild traumatic brain injury* are often used interchangeably; however, to be specific, *concussion* is a term relating to the neurological and cognitive effects of a mild TBI. A concussion occurs when the brain undergoes a violent impact injury which temporarily disrupts brain activity. The hallmarks of concussion are confusion and amnesia, which may occur immediately after the blow or several minutes later and can last from minutes to days to months, depending on the severity of the concussion. Symptoms may also include disorientation, dizziness, poor balance, disrupted attention, uncoordinated hand-eye movements, and sometimes a short period of unconsciousness. As a result of a concussion, some children may become dazed or confused while others will exhibit more serious symptoms, such as recurring headaches, repeated vomiting, seizures, and disrupted cognition. Symptoms of concussion are most often temporary and children usually recover to pre-injury functioning within a week or two.

In rare cases, the effects of a concussion can last many months or years, although the exact mechanism that causes this is not well understood and likely includes a psychological component. When symptoms last longer than a few days, the child may be experiencing *post-concussive syndrome*.

Moderate Traumatic Brain Injury

A moderate traumatic brain injury can result from an injury in which there is a loss of consciousness lasting from a few minutes to several hours. The disruption in functioning is qualitatively similar to that of a concussion, although the severity is greater as is the persistence of the symptoms. The type and degree of deficits will vary greatly based on the age of the child, the location of the injury, and other secondary factors, such as swelling or bleeding. Children who sustain a moderate TBI often experience a good recovery, especially if they have therapeutic intervention and rehabilitation, accommodations and resource services at school, and a good support network of family and friends.

TBIs are generally considered moderate if the patient exhibits one or more of the following features.

- loss of consciousness from 30 minutes to several hours

- Glasgow Coma Scale score of 9 to 12

- physical trauma evident on neuroimaging (e.g., contusions, bleeds, swelling)

- length of hospitalization due to brain-related problems is greater than 48 hours

- altered mental status involving behavioral and cognitive functioning (e.g., confusion, disorientation, irritability, depression)

- disrupted neurological functioning (e.g., vertigo, dizziness, nausea, poor balance, seizures, double-vision, headaches, sleep disturbance)

- difficulty remembering the time directly preceding the injury (*retrograde amnesia*) with disrupted ability to consolidate and recall new information after the injury (***post-traumatic amnesia***) for more than an hour

- disruption of executive functioning for weeks to months and, in rare cases, permanently (depending on the severity and location of the injury)

- fatigue or lethargy lasting weeks or months, and, in rare cases, permanently (depending on the severity and location of the injury)

Severe Traumatic Brain Injury

A severe traumatic brain injury can result from an injury in which there is a prolonged period of unconsciousness or coma lasting weeks, months, or years. A child who remains unconscious for years can be described as being in a deep coma, in a prolonged vegetative state, or in a minimally conscious state. In approximately one-third of children with a severe TBI, there is no immediate loss of consciousness. These children experience a brief lucid period during which they can communicate prior to deterioration into a comatose state.

The type and degree of deficits will vary based on the child's age, the location of injury, and secondary factors, such as swelling or bleeding. Physical, cognitive, and/or behavioral disruption may last for years with most children experiencing some degree of persistent impairment. Children with a severe TBI may never recover to the point of being independently functional, although most children achieve a sufficient level of recovery to allow them to return to school with support services. Inpatient and outpatient rehabilitative therapy and accommodations for deficits can facilitate a child's transition back to his home and his educational and recreational environments. A good support network of family and friends will also aid in the child's recovery.

Most deaths from traumatic brain injury result from severe TBIs and are generally related to compromised respiration, excessive brain swelling and herniation, seizures, hypoxia, or other medical complications.

TBIs are generally considered severe if the patient exhibits one or more of the following features.

- loss of consciousness lasting from many days to years

- Glasgow Coma Scale score of 3 to 8

- physical trauma evident on neuroimaging (e.g., contusions, bleeds, swelling)

- length of hospitalization due to brain-related problems lasts weeks to months

- retrograde amnesia with post-traumatic amnesia which may last for weeks or months

- rehabilitative therapy required

- disrupted neurological and cognitive functioning persisting for weeks to months, with subtle limitations that are often permanent

Be cautious when working with children who are in a comatose, a prolonged-vegetative, or a minimally-conscious state. A child may appear to be aware of his surroundings because midbrain functioning and brain stem reflexes can make it seem as though the child is aroused and alert to his environment. For example, the palm reflex will result in a patient squeezing one's hand, and superior colliculus reflexes can result in a patient looking toward or inconsistently tracking objects and people in the room. These and other reflex-based behaviors are often interpreted by family and even clinical professionals as evidence that the child is awake and aware of his surroundings. The child may be alert, but he is demonstrating behaviors that are automatic and unconscious and he has no awareness of what is going on around him.

It is also important to distinguish a child who is in a comatose, a minimally-conscious, or a persistent vegetative state from a child whose cognition is intact but who is unable to respond due to a variety of neuromuscular problems. For example:

- Damage to the *dopaminergic pathways* (neural pathways which transmit dopamine from one region of the brain to another) can cause *akinetic mutism*, a condition in which the child may have few, if any, body movements and no spontaneous speech. Sometimes, however, speech can be elicited and the child can track and visually orient to objects or look toward something in response to a command.

- *Locked-in syndrome* can result from damage to the ventral pons or medulla. It results in a child being unable to move or talk (i.e., quadriparetic and mute), although he may have functional cognitive abilities and be able to move his eyes purposefully.

Case Example 3 *Mark*

Dr. Lebby treated a 17-year-old adolescent named Mark who was thought to be in a comatose state following a severe brain injury due to a motor vehicle accident. Mark was transferred to the rehabilitation unit so that his parents could be trained to care for him when he was discharged. A reclining wheelchair was designed for Mark to fully support him so he could be moved around the unit and not be confined to his bed.

On a warm day, Dr. Lebby wheeled Mark outside to the rehabilitation courtyard. Mark was wearing shorts, which reminded Dr. Lebby about a recent summer day when his young nephew touched one of his legs and said, "Furry like a dog." When Dr. Lebby told Mark the story he began to smile, indicating that he may have understood Dr. Lebby's humorous comment. Dr. Lebby asked Mark to smile to indicate *yes* and remain still to indicate *no*. Using this technique, Dr. Lebby determined that Mark was not comatose, but rather presented with locked-in syndrome.

Usually, patients with locked-in syndrome can volitionally move their eyes or blink; however, due to Mark's cranial nerve injuries, he was unable to move his eyes (another symptom which made it appear that Mark was in a coma). Mark's story exemplifies how an absence of responding to the environment may not be due to deficient cognitive functioning, but related to the lack of physical ability to move or respond to stimulation.

Multiple Traumatic Brain Injuries

The effects of multiple TBIs can be considered as cumulative, in that each additional injury results in increased damage to the brain. Because the cells that are lost following a TBI are never replaced, multiple injuries can result in a gradual decline in the number of brain cells, with an expected decline in cognitive and neurological functioning. *Dementia pugilistica* is a term that is used to describe a type of dementia resulting from multiple concussions caused when boxers are repeatedly knocked out during their matches. A similar problem is seen in children who have sustained multiple brain injuries. Each additional injury has a greater effect on the child than it would have had if he had not incurred the previous injuries. Therefore, it is extremely important that a child recovering from a TBI avoids activities that place him at risk for additional injury.

Second Impact Syndrome

Second impact syndrome can occur when a child sustains a second TBI before the symptoms of the first head injury have resolved. Following a concussion, there is a period of change in brain functioning that lasts approximately one day to two weeks. If the child sustains a second concussion during this time period, the risk of more severe or permanent brain injury increases. The risk of second impact syndrome declines rapidly after the two-week period, but it can persist for many weeks or months depending on the severity of the first injury.

A child who has physical injuries, paralysis, or is unsteady on his feet due to TBI has a greater risk of falling and sustaining a second injury. Children with such difficulties require close adult supervision to minimize the risk of falling. Second impact syndrome is most commonly experienced in children and adolescents who are involved in sports. In sports-related concussive injuries, most children who experience an initial concussion can recover completely, as long as they do not return to contact sports too soon. The risk of second impact syndrome is being used to justify the increasing practice of preventing athletes from returning to competitive sports for approximately two weeks following a concussion.

Non-Accidental Trauma

Non-accidental trauma (NAT) describes injuries that are caused on purpose, such as abuse. The American Academy of Pediatrics reports that physical abuse is the leading cause of serious head injury and fatality in infants. This is also the finding at our hospital, Children's Hospital Central California, where NAT has become the most common cause of brain injury and death in infants under the age of one year. Approximately 25 percent to 30 percent of infants admitted to the hospital for NAT eventually die from their injuries. Up to 75 percent of infants diagnosed with NAT are disabled in some way for life.

NAT is one of the few ways that an infant can become severely injured from physical trauma. The use of approved safety seats in motor vehicles has reduced the number of injuries to infants. Also, a baby who falls several feet, which is consistent with a fall from a parent's arms, rarely will sustain a severe brain injury. Thus, TBIs which are not caused by motor vehicle accidents or by falls from an excessive height suggest a non-accidental cause of injury.

A baby with brain damage looks and acts like most other babies since babies have limited physical and cognitive abilities; however, many infants who appear to have good early recovery from NAT often have significant deficits in later development and functioning. As the baby develops, he may not meet expected early developmental milestones. He may also show deficits from his injury later in life when he would be expected to develop the skills served by the damaged brain regions.

Shaken Baby Syndrome

Shaken baby syndrome (SBS) is the primary cause of brain injury in non-accidental traumas and is the result of a violent criminal act. A baby does not have the ability to support his head due to its size and relatively weak neck muscles. When someone shakes a baby, the baby's head swings back and forth without control. This movement distorts and tears the soft brain tissue and crushes it against the bony structures of the skull. Blood vessels tear and cause bleeding outside of the brain and within the brain tissue.

Early CT scans often show little damage from SBS other than some swelling. Later scans can show severe brain swelling and eventually atrophy of brain tissue when the damaged cells die, causing the brain to shrivel in size.

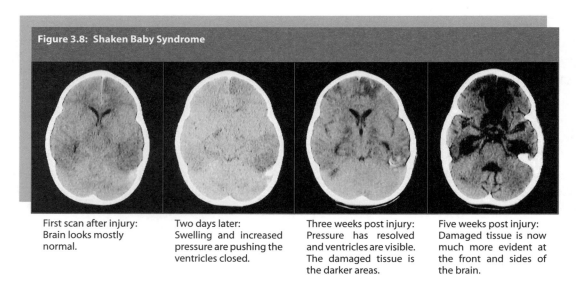

Figure 3.8: Shaken Baby Syndrome

| First scan after injury: Brain looks mostly normal. | Two days later: Swelling and increased pressure are pushing the ventricles closed. | Three weeks post injury: Pressure has resolved and ventricles are visible. The damaged tissue is the darker areas. | Five weeks post injury: Damaged tissue is now much more evident at the front and sides of the brain. |

Often the shaking force is strong enough to tear the tiny blood vessels in the eye (*retinal hemorrhages*), with 80 percent of cases showing some retinal damage. Retinal bleeding can be severe enough to cause permanent blindness. Evidence of retinal hemorrhage without a history of severe head trauma strongly suggests SBS since there are few other ways an infant can acquire such an injury.

Medical Complications

Brain injuries can cause many medical complications. The most common problems are intracranial bleeding/hemorrhaging, disrupted blood flow, intracranial swelling, disrupted autoregulation, seizures, and hypermetabolism. These medical complications have been collectively termed *secondary processes*, as the damage that results from them is not directly related to the injury, but is due to secondary mechanisms that result in additional injury to the brain.

Physical Trauma to Blood Vessels

Intracranial Bleeding/Hemorrhaging

Tearing of blood vessels causes bleeding inside the brain, or *hemorrhaging*, and can result in cell death due to loss of oxygen. Cell death can be life-threatening if it involves critical areas of the brain. A bleed can be classified as an epidural hematoma, a subdural hematoma, or an intraparenchymal (intracerebral) hematoma.

▶ **Epidural Hematoma**

An *epidural hematoma* is a buildup of blood occurring between the dura and the skull. Epidural hematomas cause more blood to leak out but less tissue damage than a subdural hematoma.

Epidural hematomas are often caused by a skull fracture which cuts a blood vessel next to the skull. The bleed forms a lens-shaped collection of blood as it pushes the dura away from the skull. Epidural hematomas can take hours to form, causing delayed symptoms.

The epidural hematoma is potentially life-threatening because the buildup of blood can result in increased pressure on the brain. The pressure can push the brain down, squeezing critical structures through the *foramen magnum* (the hole at the base of the skull) where the spinal cord connects to the brain. The pressure at the base of the brain can result in the loss of critical functions, such as breathing.

▶ **Subdural Hematoma**

A *subdural hematoma* is a bleed between the brain and the dura. Most subdural hematomas are the result of strong shearing forces acting on the brain and the meninges. These forces cause the tearing of bridging blood vessels between the dura and the brain, as well as the shearing of blood vessels within the brain tissue. Under the hematoma, there is often damage to the nerve axons.

Subdural hematomas usually result in less bleeding but generally cause more injury to the brain tissue. The prognosis for a subdural hematoma is worse than that for an epidural hematoma.

▶ **Intraparenchymal (Intracerebral) Hematoma**

An *intraparenchymal (intracerebral) hematoma* is an accumulation of blood within the tissue of the brain (*parenchyma*), often associated with contusions or tearing of the brain. When the force of an injury is strong enough to tear blood vessels, it is also strong enough to tear axons because they are more fragile than blood vessels. The presence of *petechial hemorrhages* (tiny spots of blood) on a brain scan indicates that there was tearing of tiny blood vessels within the brain. When blood is found in the ventricular system, the injury is generally very serious and the prognosis for recovery is poor.

Autoregulation

Autoregulation is a process in which the blood vessels expand or constrict to regulate pressure inside the brain. In a healthy brain, this mechanism keeps the blood pressure inside the brain constant even though the blood pressure for the body changes. A TBI disrupts autoregulation. This means that changes in the body's blood pressure will affect brain blood pressure. The result is damage to brain cells due to a reduction in oxygenated blood flow (*hypoxia*) or damage to the brain's vessels and cells due to too much pressure.

Damage or Disruption to Blood Vessels and Blood Flow

The physical force of trauma to the brain can result in damage to the blood vessels. Dr. Lebby treated a young child who had sustained a TBI, resulting in a fracture to the base of his skull. The child presented with symptoms that were more consistent with a stroke than a diffuse brain injury. After reviewing the brain scans, it became apparent that the child had no blood flow through his left internal carotid artery, the main vessel that supplies blood to most of the left side of the brain. The skull fracture had damaged the internal carotid artery where it entered the brain, causing the child to suffer significant damage due to the disruption of blood supply (*ischemia*), but not due to the actual physical trauma to the brain.

Blood vessels are often thought of as passive tubes through which blood flows in (arteries) and out (veins) of the brain. The vascular system, however, is more accurately described as an organ system of the body, with functioning that is often disrupted by TBI. For example, TBI can disrupt blood vessel functioning resulting in the vessels constricting abnormally (*vasospasm*) or expanding in size (*vasodilation*).

An infant who had both a TBI and disruption of his blood vessel functioning demonstrated good recovery for a day or two after his TBI, but then started to rapidly decline in neurological functioning. Review of his MRI/MRA scans indicated that his right and left middle and anterior cerebral arteries had gone into spasm, cutting off the blood supply to most of his cortex. (See Figure 3.9.) The lack of blood perfusion resulted in profound injury (*ischemic encephalopathy*) to a large area of cortex which was most evident on the left side of his brain, but also apparent in his right hemisphere. (See Figure 3.10.)

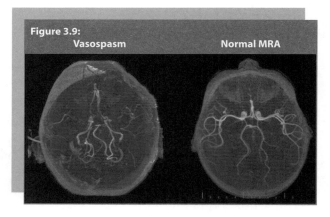

Figure 3.9: Vasospasm — Normal MRA

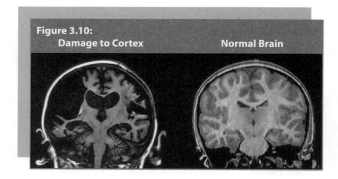

Figure 3.10: Damage to Cortex — Normal Brain

Damage to a main blood vessel due to a TBI usually results in hypoxic disruption to only one side of the brain. Different blood vessels supply each hemisphere, so blood going to one side of the brain does not normally travel across to the other hemisphere. (See Figure 3.11.)

Damage to only one vessel may not result in significant hypoxic injury. This is because the circle of Willis can allow other vessels to provide blood to the area of the brain that the damaged vessel originally supplied. (See Case Example 4.)

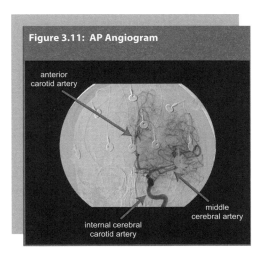

Figure 3.11: AP Angiogram

anterior carotid artery

internal cerebral carotid artery

middle cerebral artery

Case Example 4 *Braden*

Braden, a four-year-old, was accidentally backed over by an SUV and sustained a skull fracture. The injury caused damage to his right internal carotid artery where it passed through the base of the skull; however, Braden showed no signs of a stroke or of reduced blood supply to the area of the brain supplied by the right internal carotid artery. This was because the circle of Willis allowed other blood vessels to supply blood to his right middle and right anterior cerebral arteries. Specifically, the anterior communicating artery supplied blood to the anterior cerebral artery and the posterior communicating artery supplied blood to the right middle cerebral artery.

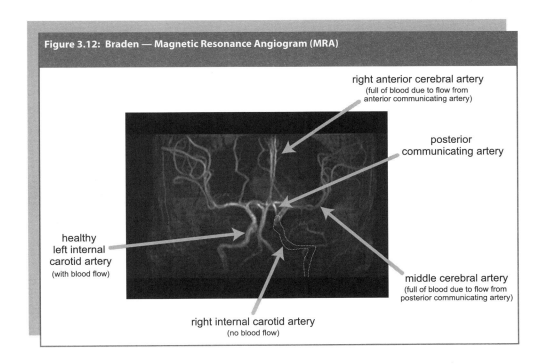

Figure 3.12: Braden — Magnetic Resonance Angiogram (MRA)

right anterior cerebral artery (full of blood due to flow from anterior communicating artery)

posterior communicating artery

healthy left internal carotid artery (with blood flow)

middle cerebral artery (full of blood due to flow from posterior communicating artery)

right internal carotid artery (no blood flow)

Intracranial Swelling

TBIs often disrupt the blood-brain barrier. Cells of the blood vessels in the brain sit so tightly together that only a few substances can pass through them. After a brain injury, the vessels may lose their ability to control fluid flow, which allows extra fluid to be released into the brain. This release of fluid is called *vasogenic edema* and it results in brain swelling. Damaged brain cells also swell, just like the cells in your thumb when they are hit by a hammer. The swelling of damaged cells is called *cytotoxic edema*. These two types of swelling increase the amount of fluid in the brain, which makes the brain increase in size.

> Swelling inside the skull is like inflating a tractor inner tube while it is in a tractor tire. Pressure inside the tire builds up slowly until the inner tube hits the inside surface of the tire. Once that happens, the pressure required to inflate the tube builds up very quickly as the tube pushes against the hard rubber of the tire.

When the brain swells, it has very little room to expand. Initially, the swelling does not cause a big increase in intracranial pressure because the ventricles absorb the extra fluid. As the fluid buildup increases, however, the spaces inside the cranial vault fill up, squeezing the ventricles and other cavities shut. The pressure within the brain begins to build rapidly.

The increased swelling can put pressure on the third cranial nerve, which causes *pupillary dilation* (large unreactive pupils) and *ptosis* (drooping eyelids). These are both signs that the pressure is becoming critical and brain herniation is imminent. *Brain herniation* is when brain tissue is pushed through a hole or across a membrane, such as dura. Increased swelling can be life-threatening if the pressure pushes the brain stem down through the *foramen magnum*, the large hole in the base of the skull through which the spinal cord passes.

If the pressure within the skull (intracranial pressure [ICP]) becomes greater than the child's blood pressure, there will be a loss of blood flow to critical brain structures. The loss of blood flow through the brain results in some areas being deprived of oxygen. Loss of oxygenated blood can cause severe hypoxic injury or even death.

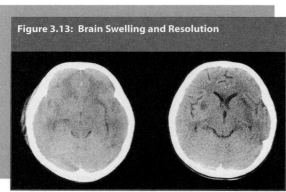

Figure 3.13: Brain Swelling and Resolution

The brain on the left has swollen to fill the entire skull, squeezing the sides flat, making it hard to see the wrinkles (sulci and gyri) and pushing the ventricles closed. The picture on the right shows the same brain after the pressure has resolved.

Infection of the Meninges and Brain

Open head or penetrating injuries allow bacteria to contaminate the meninges, the layers of skin that surround and protect the brain. This can cause a condition called *meningitis*, which is an inflammatory infection of the meninges. If the bacteria reach the brain tissue under the meninges, the child may develop *encephalitis*, an infection of the encephalon (brain).

Hydrocephalus

A TBI can disrupt the flow of cerebral spinal fluid (CSF), causing pressure to build up within the ventricles. The ventricles become dilated, expanding like balloons being filled with liquid. This condition is known as *hydrocephalus* and can become life-threatening if pressure builds up to critical levels. Hydrocephalus can result from meningitis. It can also result from conditions that block the flow of CSF, such as physical displacement of brain tissue, fractures, hematomas, or foreign objects from penetrating injuries. Figure 3.14 shows three views of normal ventricles (top pictures) and hydrocephalus (bottom pictures).

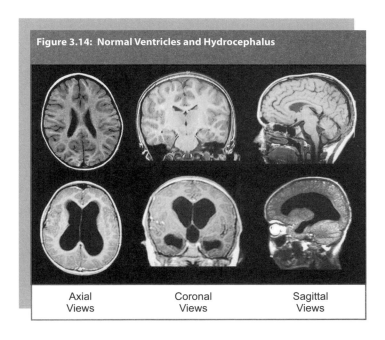

Figure 3.14: Normal Ventricles and Hydrocephalus

Axial Views   Coronal Views   Sagittal Views

Seizures

Brain injuries increase the risk of seizures. Some seizures can be life-threatening and others may just disrupt functioning for a short time. Up to half of all children with penetrating injuries or intracranial bleeds will have seizures. Only 5 percent of children with TBIs that do not involve penetration or bleeding will have complications from seizures.

Most seizures occur within a short time after an injury, but they can happen at any time. The more time that passes after an injury, the less likely the child with have post-traumatic seizures. Seizures increase the metabolic activity of the brain and can result in additional cell death due to a loss of oxygen (i.e., *hypoxic-ischemic injury*). In addition, seizures can increase intracranial pressure, resulting in some of the complications mentioned earlier in this chapter.

Hypermetabolism

Nutrition is critically important in a child with a head injury. TBI can increase the metabolic demands of the brain by 30 percent to 60 percent. Feeding difficulties may compound the problem. Some children can lose as much as a fifth of their body weight within the first few weeks of their hospitalization. As a result of metabolic changes, increased demands for nutrition, and feeding difficulties associated with TBI, patients are routinely referred for an evaluation and follow-up care by a dietician.

Appendix 3A: Common Symptoms Associated with Areas of Brain Damage

Damage to various areas of the brain can cause problems as listed below.

▶ **Frontal Lobes**
- Broca's (expressive or motor) aphasia—the inability to produce fluent speech; speech is labored and is often choppy with few words (telegraphic)
- verbal (oral-motor) apraxia—difficulty sequencing movements to produce speech and control the muscles of the mouth
- paralysis (loss of motor function) on the side opposite the damage
- apathy syndrome—a loss of self-initiation, drive, or self-directed behavior
- disrupted executive functioning—deficits with higher-order cognitive skills
- problems regulating behavior in different environments
- trouble controlling emotions
- disrupted social and interpersonal functioning; impaired ability to relate to others
- difficulty sustaining attention

▶ **Temporal Lobes**
- amnesia—more commonly anterograde (inability to store new memories) but can also affect retrieval of old memories (retrograde)
- auditory agnosia—loss of the ability to interpret sounds (verbal and nonverbal)
- pure word deafness—loss of the ability to understand words but without the loss of the ability to recognize or identify nonverbal sounds
- instinctive drives—difficulties regulating instinctive behaviors, such as fear, aggression, and sexual and feeding behaviors
- Wernicke's (sensory or receptive) aphasia—a deficit involving the comprehension or understanding of language (dominant hemisphere)
- receptive aprosody—the inability to understand prosody, such as the interpretation of intonation or the emotional content communicated by the tone of a voice (non-dominate hemisphere)

▶ **Parietal Lobes**
- loss of sensation correlating to the specific area of sensory cortex
- attentional neglect—inability to attend to objects or space opposite the hemisphere injured
- difficulties solving problems requiring visual-spatial processing (non-dominant hemisphere)
- agnosia syndromes—visual agnosia (occipital-parietal); auditory agnosia (temporal-parietal); somatosensory agnosia, also called astereognosis (superior-parietal); simultaneous agnosia or difficulty perceiving two objects at the same time (bilateral occipital-parietal)
- alexia—disruption of previously learned reading skills
- agraphia—disruption of writing skills
- acalculia—disruption of mathematics/arithmetic skills
- construction apraxia—disruption of the ability to construct 3D block designs when matching pictures of models

▶ **Occipital Lobes**
- loss of visual perception for areas of the visual field that correspond to the damaged cortex
- difficulty processing complex visual information

▶ **Cerebellum**
- ataxia—loss of motor coordination
- dysarthria—neuromotor difficulty in articulation and voicing
- loss of muscle tone causing child to become floppy, appearing like a rag doll
- loss of balance when moving
- poor ability to coordinate muscle movements
- dysmetria—overshooting when trying to make precise movements
- intention tremor—tremor that occurs with volitional movements and often becomes worse as a movement reaches its goal
- nystagmus—tracking of the eyes that is jerky
- disrupted cognitive processing involving attention, language, memory, social awareness, and intellect

▶ **Thalamus**
- loss of functioning relating to the specific pathways that are damaged
- hypersensitivity or sensory defensiveness

▶ **Hypothalamus**
- poor control of internal bodily states, such as temperature, hunger, and thirst
- hormonal imbalance affecting growth, puberty, behavior, and emotions
- disrupted autonomic nervous system function involving the fight-or-flight response, sexual behavior, etc.

▶ **Limbic System**
- emotional disorders involving pleasure, depression, anxiety, fear, etc.
- amnesia for new learning (anterograde) and difficulties with retrieval of old memories (retrograde)
- disrupted primitive emotional drives involving aggression, sexual and predatory behaviors, etc.
- disrupted instinctive behaviors involving dominance-submission, approach-avoidance for mating and fighting, etc.

▶ **Midbrain**
- loss of consciousness or disrupted arousal
- coma
- disrupted ability to maintain wakefulness or cognitive arousal
- disrupted sleep patterns
- disrupted attention
- disrupted ability to orient to visual or auditory stimuli
- changes in normal muscle tone
- changes in pain responses to stimuli

▶ **Brain Stem**
- loss of life-sustaining functions, such as breathing and heartbeat regulation
- loss of consciousness
- loss of communication between the brain and spinal cord, resulting in conditions such as paralysis
- changes in muscle tone
- disrupted reflexive movements of the eyes
- disrupted reflexive movements of the mouth for swallowing, coughing, vomiting, sneezing, etc.
- poor control of body temperature

Chapter 4

TBI-Related Language Disorders

▌Communication

Communication is much more than spoken or written words. For many years, Dr. Lebby has defined *communication* as "the ability to change what someone else is thinking." Dr. Lebby's definition implies that communication is more than just getting your thoughts across to others. It involves the active process of influencing someone else's thoughts and behaviors. Communication involves both verbal language and nonverbal behaviors.

This chapter describes a variety of language-based disorders, including conditions that involve aspects of both verbally- and nonverbally-based communication. (See Appendix 4A, page 85, for a glossary of language-based disorders.)

Verbal Language

Verbal language is the phonetic message that ultimately relates to the words we hear. Language is made up of surface structure and deep structure. *Surface structure* corresponds to the actual words spoken. *Deep structure* is the underlying meaning of the sentence, or the speaker's message. A speaker communicates deep structure using words and prosody.

Prosody is the melody, rhythm, and inflection of speech. Prosody helps to clarify the message when the surface structure is ambiguous. When a speaker uses prosody, a phrase with more than one meaning can be accurately interpreted by the listener. For example, *It's hot today?* has a different meaning than *It's hot today!* Although the words are the same, the first one is a question and the second one is an exclamation. Disorders of prosody can relate to the expression of prosody (*expressive aprosodia*) or the understanding of prosody (*receptive aprosodia*).

Other aspects of language that are important in clarifying the deep structure or intent of the message include the *syntax* (rules that dictate how words are combined) and the *semantics* (correct use of words to portray a specific meaning).

Nonverbal Behaviors

In addition to spoken words, nonverbal behaviors, such as body movements, eye contact, tone of voice, and speed/rate of speech, enhance the communication of a message. When people interact, they rely on nonverbal behaviors to help them express their ideas to others and to understand the messages others communicate to them.

TBI-Related Communication Deficits

TBI can cause disorders of communication without disrupting language or can cause disorders of language without disrupting communication. For example, a child may lose the ability to talk but retain the ability to communicate via other modalities (e.g., oral-motor apraxia). Another child may lose the ability to communicate his thoughts but retain the ability to articulate (e.g., Wernicke's-type aphasia). The type of communication deficit depends on the location and severity of the brain damage. (See Appendix 4B, page 86, for a list of the areas of the brain that are involved with language functioning.)

After a TBI, the surface and deep structure of a communicated message may not match. For example, a child may wish to express the message *I'm hungry* but the words he uses do not communicate this message. The problem in communicating the deep structure may be related to the wrong choice of words, poor sentence structure, paraphasic or neologistic errors (phoneme, syllable, or word substitution), perseveration, or other pathological utterances in addition to disrupted prosody.

Due to expressive language or communication problems, an injured child's verbal responses may not accurately reflect his knowledge. The child may understand the information and have the ability to conceptualize his response mentally but be unable to efficiently explain his ideas. When asked a question, a child with TBI may talk too much or too little. He may circumlocute, that is give long answers that include a lot of words but little, if any, relevant content and may even miss the point altogether. On the other hand, he may give short answers that do not contain enough information to answer the question.

Receptive language deficits are often evident in children recovering from TBI. Some children with TBI-related verbal/auditory processing deficits experience a problem that is similar to listening to someone who speaks English rapidly with a strong foreign accent. The child spends so much time trying to decipher the person's speech that he fails to fully process the verbal information. This results in poor understanding, difficulty attending to the speaker, and a disrupted ability to remember information.

An injured child may retain the ability to respond with gestures, facial expressions, and body movements. Because of this ability, his family and teachers may overestimate his comprehension of conversations and his ability to communicate. Unfortunately, the child may not fully understand all of the information they present to him, especially complex questions, statements, or communications. The case example on the next page demonstrates how easily a child's language functioning can be overestimated by just a few correct responses.

Case Example 1 *Natasha*

Natasha, a 14-year-old, was involved in a car accident and sustained a severe brain injury. The medical reports indicated that she had intact language functioning, even with damage to her left hemisphere. We thought that Natasha must have some language functioning in her right hemisphere because the severity of the injury to her left hemisphere would normally have resulted in an aphasia syndrome (loss of language function).

When we first examined Natasha, we asked questions, such as *What is your name?*, *Where are we?*, and *What is this building?* Natasha did not answer; she just nodded. We asked, "Are you in any pain?" Natasha nodded. We asked, "Is your name Natasha?" Again, she nodded. We then asked, "Are you an elephant?" and "Are we on the moon?" Natasha nodded to both of these questions as well.

It quickly became clear that Natasha was nodding to all questions but had no idea what we were asking her. The physician intern who wrote in the chart that she had intact language must have only asked close-ended questions that required affirmative responses, such as *Are you 14 years old?* Natasha likely nodded to each question and the doctor assumed she understood what he was asking her.

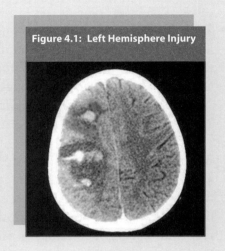

Figure 4.1: Left Hemisphere Injury

Left Hemisphere Versus Right Hemisphere Language Processing

In most people, the left hemisphere, generally referred to as the *dominant hemisphere*, houses the ability to formulate and comprehend language; however, in a very small number of people language ability is found in the right hemisphere. Left versus right hemisphere dominance for language can vary, especially for children who sustained a TBI early in life or who have long-standing neurological problems, such as epilepsy. The brains of young children with brain damage to the dominant hemisphere (usually the left) can go through a process of restructuring. The change in brain structure (*plasticity*) can allow for the non-dominant hemisphere (usually the right) to take over some of the functions that were localized in the damaged dominant hemisphere. This process of plasticity can allow a child with damage to the dominant hemisphere to regain some of the lost language functions.

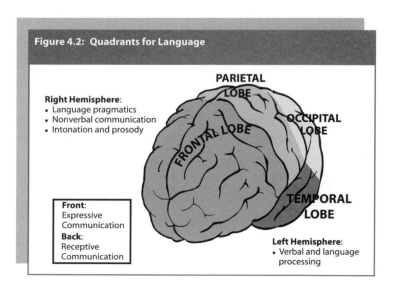

Figure 4.2: Quadrants for Language

Right Hemisphere:
- Language pragmatics
- Nonverbal communication
- Intonation and prosody

PARIETAL LOBE

FRONTAL LOBE

OCCIPITAL LOBE

TEMPORAL LOBE

Front: Expressive Communication
Back: Receptive Communication

Left Hemisphere:
- Verbal and language processing

Handedness has also been shown to affect the degree to which language is lateralized in the brain. Children who are left-handed have a higher prevalence of right hemisphere language processing than children who are right-handed. You should not assume, however, that a left-handed child has atypical language dominance (right hemisphere) because approximately 90 percent of children who are left-handed will still have left hemisphere dominance for language.

> **M**yth: If the left hemisphere is severely injured, the right hemisphere will take over language functions and the child will be fine.
>
> **F**act: The right hemisphere can take over language function in neonates and very young infants to some degree. With older children and adolescents, however, this is much less likely and long-term problems with language are common.

Damage to the Language Dominant Hemisphere

Damage to the language cortex in the dominant hemisphere can cause a disorder of verbal communication called *aphasia*. Aphasia disrupts language functioning and can range from mild word-finding difficulties to a global loss of receptive and expressive language ability. Often when injuries are localized to the dominant hemisphere, the nonverbal aspects of language are preserved (e.g., prosody, intonation, body language).

Damage to the Non-Language Dominant Hemisphere

The *non-dominant hemisphere* controls prosodic processing. Injuries to the non-dominant hemisphere may disrupt language pragmatics or nonverbal communication (*aprosody*), which can make it difficult for the child to communicate effectively.

In addition, damage to either hemisphere at the front of the brain can disrupt expressive communication, while damage to either hemisphere toward the back of the brain can disrupt receptive communication.

Damage to Both Hemispheres

In general, most children with brain injuries have some form of diffuse damage which affects both hemispheres. Diffuse damage also frequently affects the frontal lobes, which can lead to difficulty with communication due to disruption of the following functions.

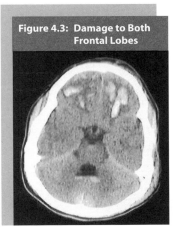

Figure 4.3: Damage to Both Frontal Lobes

- attention (focus on conversation)
- multitasking
- executive functioning
- processing speed
- social-communication (pragmatics)
  - grasping another's perspective
  - interpreting humor or complex language, such as innuendo or sarcasm

69

- maintaining a theme within a conversation
- taking turns in conversation or in play
- thinking of comments to sustain a discussion
- interpreting what others say (disruption can result in the child acting inappropriately)
- participating in group conversations (the extra time it takes the child to figure out the point to a conversation can make him appear different to his friends)
- responding to nonverbal cues that normally let others know when to stop a conversation, change a topic, stop a behavior, or add a comment
- inhibiting responses (disruption results in frequent interruption of others)
- listening vigilance (disruption results in daydreaming or talking instead of listening)
- refraining from making comments that he thinks are cute or funny, but are actually annoying to others

---

Case Example 2 *Nicholas*

Nicholas was 11 years old when he was involved in a motor vehicle accident. He recovered relatively well from his brain injury, but he was still having difficulty with language processing a year later.

Nicholas's case was interesting because he loved to laugh and tell jokes. Nicholas continued to tell jokes after his injury although his ability to do so was disrupted. Even though he knew the words to the jokes, the timing and rhythm of his speech was slow, causing his friends to lose interest or become distracted. Also, Nicholas could not emphasize the right parts of the joke, so his friends didn't realize when he had said the punch line. When someone told him a joke, Nicholas had difficulty integrating all of the information quickly enough to "get it," even though the joke was at an appropriate developmental level.

As in Nicholas's case, mild language disorders may disrupt a child's ability to socialize. He may become uncomfortable in social situations because he doesn't fit in or because friends stop including him in conversations or games. Children with mild language disorders tend to be seen as less knowledgeable or friendly but often just need encouragement and extra time.

Dysnomia

Dysnomia is a marked difficulty in retrieving nouns or words needed for oral or written language. Word-finding and verbal formulation deficits are common in children with TBI. Children often compensate for word-finding problems by using phrases, such as *that thing*, associated words (e.g., saying *pencil* instead of *pen*), and gestures instead of using the actual object name. They may also hesitate or use fillers, such as *hmmm, errr,* or *um,* to give them time to think of the word they want to use. Their vocabulary development may be slower than expected and can result in delayed language development and reduced confidence in their language skills. Language deficits are often mistaken for shyness, withdrawal, or depression.

The Source for TBI – Children & Adolescents　　　70

Paraphasic or Neologistic Errors

After a brain injury, a child's language may include strange remarks or words, known as *paraphasic* or *neologistic errors*. Most of the time, the child will not be aware that these utterances are incorrect or inappropriate. Paraphasic errors are classified as being either verbal or literal, based on the type of error the child produces. Neologisms are errors of speech involving the expression of nonwords.

1. *Verbal paraphasia* is when the child substitutes one word for another (e.g., the child sees a chair and calls it a table). Verbal paraphasias are often semantically related.

2. *Literal*, *phonological*, or *phonemic paraphasia* is when the child produces a word that contains a phonological error. The word produced is usually similar to the word the child wishes to express but it includes a phoneme or a syllable substitution (e.g., the child says *cabera* instead of *camera*).

3. *Neologisms* are word-like utterances that are expressed and sound like real words, but are not real words (e.g., *rockside*).

Aphasia Syndromes

Aphasia is a loss or an impairment of the ability to produce and/or comprehend language. Usually aphasias are the result of damage to the language centers of the brain, which are almost always located in the left hemisphere. The type and severity of aphasia depends on the following.

- location of the injury (most important factor)
- severity of the injury
- extent or size of the injury

> In general, frontal damage causes problems with expressive speech (Broca's-type aphasia). Posterior damage causes problems with the understanding of language (Wernicke's-type aphasia). Damage that involves most of the hemisphere can cause global aphasia.

Broca's-Type Aphasia

Note: We prefer to use the term *Broca's-type aphasia* (versus Broca's aphasia) as it describes the type of aphasia but does not necessarily imply damage to Broca's area.

Key Feature ▶ problems involving the production of speech

Broca's-type aphasia is also called *expressive*, *dysfluent*, or *motor aphasia*. It is most commonly caused by damage to the left frontal lobe, just in front and at the bottom of the primary motor cortex (a region called *Broca's area*). Expressive aphasia can be seen in patients who do not have damage to Broca's area, but damage usually involves this area or is close to it.

Patients with Broca's-type aphasia have such difficulty with expressive language skills that they typically use the fewest words necessary to communicate the message. These words are primarily nouns and verbs but can include a few grammatical functor words, such as conjunctions, articles, prepositions, and auxiliary verbs. The use of shortened utterances is called *telegraphic speech*.

Primary Symptoms

- word-finding difficulty
- paraphasic or neologistic errors
- telegraphic speech
- poor sentence structure (syntax)
- effortful and slow speech that is often halting
- abnormal inflection, rhythm, and intonation/melodic contour (prosody)
- similar errors may be found with writing (agraphia)
- poor articulation with features of apraxia and dysarthria
- abnormal repetition, which differentiates it from transcortical motor aphasia
- relatively good comprehension of speech and written language

Case Example 3 *Evelyn*

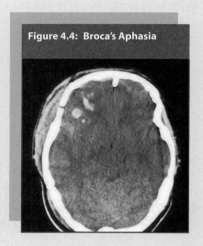

Figure 4.4: Broca's Aphasia

Evelyn, a 17-year-old, was involved in a motor vehicle accident in which she injured her left frontal lobe. Most of the damage occurred around Broca's area which resulted in a severe dysfluent aphasia syndrome. Evelyn was unable to produce fluent speech, had severe word-finding difficulty, and produced many paraphasic errors. Damage to other areas of her frontal lobes also made her perseverative (i.e., she got stuck on certain words or ideas). Evelyn had no difficulty with receptive language skills and her comprehension was fully intact.

The following is a sample of Evelyn's performance during a language-based assessment. The colored numbers represent how many seconds had passed since Evelyn began her response. Evelyn worked on each response for one minute before the examiner moved on to another picture.

The examiner shows Evelyn a picture of a birthday party scene. (Note: Evelyn perseverates on the word *using* and produces verbal paraphasias, such as *elephant* for *dog* and *bed* for *table*.)

Examiner: "What is going on in this picture?"

Evelyn: "Using … using her … **15** …. no … um … errr … party … **22** … errr … hmmm … using her thing … for that **30** … for the table … the thing … then … use a hat … **47** … and … um … hmmm … a tea … no … hmmm … elephant … no … use a bed … **60**."

Evelyn, continued

The examiner shows Evelyn a picture of a snail.

Examiner: "What is this?"

Evelyn: "You hit ...no ...you hmmm ...hit ...you hit it in the ground ...no ...**20** ...don't know ...**30**."

Examiner: "Where would you find one of these?"

Evelyn: "Hmmm ...um ...you ...you ...hmmm ...hmmm ...**45** ...you ...get it in the mud ...no ...get it in the ...oh never mind ...**60**."

Wernicke's-Type Aphasia

Note: We prefer to use the term *Wernicke's-type aphasia* (versus Wernicke's aphasia), as it describes the type of aphasia but does not necessarily imply damage to Wernicke's area.

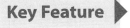 **Key Feature** ▶ problems with the extraction of the meaning of language which disrupts both understanding and expression

Wernicke's-type aphasia is also called *receptive aphasia*, *fluent aphasia*, or *sensory aphasia*. It is most commonly caused by damage within the temporal–parietal region of the language dominant hemisphere. Wernicke's-type aphasia can be seen in patients who do not have damage to Wernicke's area, but damage usually involves this area or is close to it.

Primary Symptoms
- fluent, effortless speech that is often rapid and verbose (*logorrhea*)
- disrupted comprehension for both oral and written language
- verbalizations contain little or no meaning
- paraphasic errors (literal/phonemic and verbal) and neologisms (words that aren't real)
- omissions of parts of words, whole words, or phrases
- lack of awareness of illness or deficits (*anosognosia*)
- abnormal repetition, which differentiates it from transcortical sensory aphasia
- speech with normal inflection and rhythm (*prosody*)
- correct grammar (i.e., rules for combining phonemes/words is intact)

Case Example 4 *Jack*

Jack, a 16-year-old, was involved in a motor vehicle accident. His brain injury involved the left dominant hemisphere for language. Most of the damage to Jack's brain was in Wernicke's area, which resulted in a severe fluent aphasia syndrome.

Jack had difficulty understanding others and could only understand basic questions, such as *What is this?* or *What is this used for?* Jack had lost the semantics of language and his expressive speech was also affected. He spoke fluently and had relatively good syntax, but the content of his speech did not make sense. Almost every word was a paraphasic error or a neologism. *Word salad* is a term that has been used to describe this type of aphasia. It was as if Jack took a bunch of words, put them in a bowl, tossed them like a salad, and then spoke them.

The following is a sample of Jack's performance during a language assessment.

The examiner shows a baseball cap to Jack.

Examiner: "What is this?"
Jack: "It's a blue rockside."

Examiner: "A blue rockside?"
Jack: "Yes."

Examiner: "What is a blue rockside?"
Jack: "Something you write with, to draw."

Examiner: "Show me." (Examiner handed Jack the hat.)
Jack: "You write with it." (Jack put the hat on his head.)

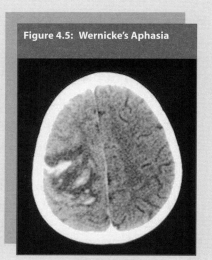

Figure 4.5: Wernicke's Aphasia

Next the examiner shows Jack a toy airplane.

Examiner: What is this?"
Jack: "Something epernevia."

Examiner: "What is it for?"
Jack: "You rub it on your belt."

Then the examiner shows Jack a picture of a kitchen scene with a mother and two children.

Examiner: "Tell me about this picture."
Jack: "Gojerra … [pause] … somebody is getting gojerra." (Jack spoke while pointing to the boy in the picture.)

"Paint sticks." (Jack pointed to the kitchen table.)

"It's a white birdcage." (Jack pointed to the chair.)

Examiner: "What is happening?" (Examiner pointed to the kitchen window.)
Jack: "Marinara."

74

Global Aphasia

Key Feature ▶ broad disruption of expressive and receptive language

The region of brain around the sylvian fissure (*perisylvian zone*) extends from the frontal lobe back to the parietal lobe and down to the temporal lobe. Damage to this area of the dominant hemisphere can disrupt both receptive and expressive language functioning.

If the brain is injured on the dominant side, swelling frequently puts pressure on the entire hemisphere of damage, resulting in disruption of most language functions. Similarly, if only the non-dominant hemisphere becomes damaged and swells, it can push against the dominant hemisphere, resulting in disrupted language processing. Generalized swelling in either hemisphere may cause global aphasia symptoms due to disruption of the cortex around the sylvian fissure. If global aphasia is caused by swelling, the aphasia symptoms usually improve quickly as the swelling resolves. If, however, there is a lot of damage to the tissue in the perisylvian region of the language dominant hemisphere, there may be much less recovery and symptoms can persist for months, years, or even indefinitely.

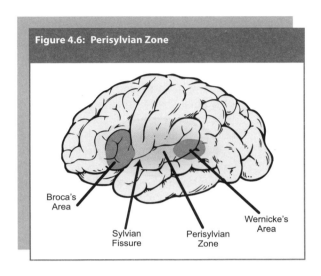

Figure 4.6: Perisylvian Zone

Broca's Area

Wernicke's Area

Sylvian Fissure

Perisylvian Zone

Primary Symptoms
- may have symptoms of both expressive and receptive aphasias
- loss of language skills can range in severity from profound to mild
- can have more difficulty with language production (fluency) than the understanding of language and vice versa
- may be mute and unable to understand symbolic language, including sign language and letter-number identification
- may express words perseveratively
- may use automatic words or phrases in inappropriate contexts
- may be unable to repeat linguistic information presented auditorily

Case Example 5 *Erin*

Erin, a 15-year-old, was the victim of a drive-by shooting. The bullet went through her left frontal lobe and traveled to her left parietal lobe. The injury was extensive and left her with damage to the entire left hemisphere around the sylvian fissure. Erin's case is extreme, but it highlights the syndrome very well. Erin's functioning over the course of her recovery was as follows.

Examination at discharge from the hospital

▶ Global aphasia
- able to produce a few short words via imitation but most were incorrectly articulated
- no ability to understand language in verbal or written form, including letters
- could not communicate her needs verbally or in written form
- unable to sequence sounds to produce words (i.e., dense verbal apraxia)

▶ Nonverbal and visual-spatial reasoning—low average for her age (Performance Intelligence Quotient [PIQ] = 82)

▶ Executive functioning—deficient on all measures

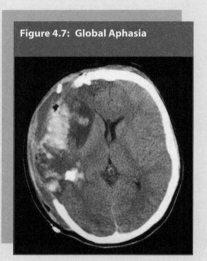

Figure 4.7: Global Aphasia

Examination six months after her injury

▶ Expressive aphasia remained severe.
- able to produce a few short words via imitation but most were incorrectly articulated
- able to say *A* and *B* when shown the letters but not name other letters or numbers
- able to count to 10 and say the alphabet to E
- no spontaneous speech

▶ Receptive aphasia had resolved a little but was still severe.
- turned when she heard her name; looked at her mother when someone said, "Mom"
- inconsistently identified colors to verbal prompts
- unable to follow single-part commands or any multi-word phrases

▶ Nonverbal and visual spatial reasoning—low average for her age (PIQ = 86)

▶ Executive functioning—had improved but remained deficient overall

Examination two years after her injury (most recovery had taken place)

▶ Expressive aphasia remained severe and Erin was functionally mute.
- able to write some basic, over-learned items (i.e., things you learn early and use so frequently that you never forget them, such as your name, the alphabet, counting to 10) but unable to write any functionally-relevant words (e.g., *pain, hurt, scared, tired, lost, home*)
- unable to produce spontaneous words; could only produce words via imitation
- unable to name letters shown to her
- able to identify (point to) the letters *A, B, C, D, E, G* when asked, but unable to read any words

▶ Receptive aphasia had only improved slightly; it was still severe.
- able to respond consistently when someone called her name
- unable to identify pictures from a field of four when given a multi-word phrase (*red table*) or follow a verbal command involving more than one word

▶ Nonverbal and visual spatial reasoning—had improved from the low average to the high average range, with the central tendency being average (PIQ = 96)

▶ Executive functioning—remained deficient, with perseveration and rigidity of thought

76

Anomic/Dysnomic Aphasia

Key Feature ▶ difficulty retrieving specific words

Damage to almost any region of the brain associated with language functioning can result in *anomic aphasia*, or word-finding difficulty. The phenomena of anomic aphasia is similar to when you are trying to think of a word and "it's on the tip of your tongue."

Anomic aphasia is very common after a TBI because word-finding is one of the most sensitive functions of the language system. Even if no other language disruption is evident, a mild injury can significantly disrupt the efficiency of word-finding. Word-finding difficulty may also be a residual deficit when the child recovers from a more serious language disorder, such as Broca's-type or Wernicke's-type aphasia.

Primary Symptoms
- word-finding difficulty
- circumlocution (talking about a word rather than using the specific/exact term)
- word-retrieval deficits despite fluent speech
- difficulties with verbal formulation

Case Example 6 *Jan*

Jan, a 17-year-old, was involved in a high-speed automobile collision. She sustained diffuse injury to her left hemisphere. The injury caused her to have language difficulties relating to word finding and motor problems with her right side.

Jan had little difficulty speaking in sentences, but she often got stuck when using nouns. She described her problem as, "I know the word I am trying to say but it is stuck in my head."

When we asked Jan to name an object, she would struggle to find the right word, become frustrated, and end up saying, "I don't know." Even though she could not name the object, she was able to choose the object's label from a list of options and describe its function. Since Jan had no difficulty recognizing the object or describing its use, it was obvious that her problem was specific to naming and not visually based.

Alexia

| Key Feature ▶ | newly-acquired illiteracy (inability to read) |

Alexia is a syndrome in which damage to the brain disrupts the child's ability to read. Alexia is different from dyslexia because alexia is a loss of previously-learned reading ability, whereas dyslexia is the failure to develop age-appropriate reading skills. The two most common forms of alexia are *pure alexia* (also called *alexia without dysgraphia*) and *alexia with dysgraphia*. *Dysgraphia* is a disorder of writing ability, caused by damage to the brain.

Primary Symptoms

- inability to read or point to specific letters or words on command
- alexia without dysgraphia results in the inability to read with the retained ability to write
- alexia with dysgraphia results in the loss of both reading and writing skills
- no difficulty copying words or letters (i.e., It is not a visual problem.)
- other language functions generally remain intact

Pure Alexia (Alexia Without Dysgraphia)

| Key Feature ▶ | newly-acquired inability to read with intact ability to write |

Pure alexia is generally caused by damage to the pathways from the visual cortex on either side of the brain to the left (or dominant) temporal/parietal area responsible for reading. The damage prevents visual information relating to letters and words from going to the part of the brain that attaches linguistic meaning to the visual information.

In pure alexia, the person loses the ability to read but does not lose the ability to write. This is because the area of the brain that controls reading is damaged, but the area that controls writing is not.

Note: Alexia without dysgraphia is considered a disconnection syndrome but because cortical damage can also cause forms of alexia, it is not included in the following section on disconnection syndromes.

78

Case Example 7 *Erin*

Erin, mentioned on page 76, had pure alexia. She was unable to read but she could write; however, because of her severe receptive aphasia, she could not write sentences spoken to her. Instead, Dr. Lebby drew several pictures on a white board (e.g., bus, cat, dog, tree) and then drew a line beside each picture. Dr. Lebby wrote the label for the first picture (e.g., *bus*). He then pointed to the other blank lines. Erin was quickly able to write the label for each picture even though later she was unable to read what she had just written.

Alexia with Dysgraphia

Key Feature ▶ newly-acquired inability to read and write

Alexia with dysgraphia is a condition where the child loses both the ability to read and to write. Alexia with dysgraphia is generally caused by damage to the left (or dominant) temporal–parietal area involving both the *angular gyrus* and *supramarginal gyrus*.

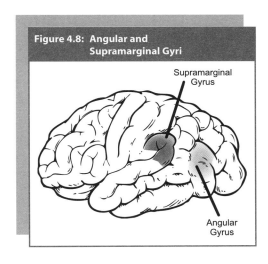

Figure 4.8: Angular and Supramarginal Gyri

Supramarginal Gyrus

Angular Gyrus

Disconnection Syndromes Causing Aphasia

The following aphasia syndromes, known as *disconnection syndromes*, are caused by damage to the communication pathways between different areas of the brain.

Conduction Aphasia

Key Feature ▶ problems repeating information

The *arcuate fasciculus* is the band of fibers that connects the posterior language areas (Wernicke's area) to the frontal speech areas (Broca's area). (See Figure 4.9, page 80.) Damage to the arcuate fasciculus prevents language-based information from traveling via this pathway, so it must use less efficient routes. This disrupts and slows the transmission of information.

Primary Symptoms

- impaired ability to repeat auditorily-presented information
- speech may contain paraphasias, but unlike Wernicke's-type aphasia, the patient may be immediately aware of any error and will try to correct it
- usually normal inflection and rhythm (prosodic contour) of speech
- often no problems with comprehension of spoken or written words
- may have problems with reading

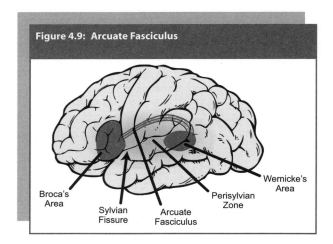

Figure 4.9: Arcuate Fasciculus

Broca's Area — Sylvian Fissure — Arcuate Fasciculus — Perisylvian Zone — Wernicke's Area

Conduction aphasias often do not significantly disrupt a child's or adolescent's ability to communicate, but they can if repetition is required, as it was in Kathy's case.

Case Example 8 *Kathy*

Kathy, a 17-year-old, had an injury to her arcuate fasciculus due to a small caliber, low velocity gunshot wound. She was able to function relatively well as long as she did not have to listen to and repeat back a lot of information.

Prior to her injury, Kathy worked part-time at a ticket counter during the weekends. As part of her job, she had to take ticket orders and repeat back the information to the customers before finalizing the sales. After she recovered, Kathy found that she was able to understand all of the information, but she was not able to process it quickly enough. She could not use her efficient pathways (arcuate fasciculus) to repeat the information back accurately. Kathy also produced some literal paraphasic errors, but these errors did not significantly disrupt her verbal communication since she was aware of them and would immediately correct them.

Pure Word Deafness

Key Feature > problems comprehending verbal language

Pure word deafness is caused by damage to Wernicke's area or by a disruption of auditory input to this region. Children with pure word deafness have receptive deficits that are restricted to speech and language. Even though they cannot comprehend speech sounds, children with pure word deafness can still recognize non-speech sounds (e.g., a dog barking) because those sounds are not processed in Wernicke's area.

Primary Symptoms

- inability to understand auditorily-presented linguistic information
- no difficulty identifying non-language-based sounds
- no difficulty speaking, reading, or writing

Children with pure word deafness are not deaf. They can hear and identify non-speech sounds without difficulty. As demonstrated by Madison, they can also recover some of their ability to understand speech by using visual cues from facial expressions and lip movements.

Case Example 9 *Madison*

Madison, a five-year-old, was injured when she fell onto concrete from a height of several feet. Madison's injury caused a small hemorrhage in the area of cortex between the auditory cortex and Wernicke's area.

Early in Madison's recovery, she responded normally to sounds in her room, but she was unable to "hear" what people said. In reality, her hearing was fine, but she did not respond to words or speech.

As Madison recovered, she began to understand speech but only when she was facing the speaker so she could use facial cues to compensate for her poor auditory comprehension skills. Eventually, Madison fully recovered her ability to understand speech when it was spoken slowly and clearly, even without visual cues. She continued to have difficulty, however, when multiple people were talking at the same time or when someone spoke quickly or did not articulate clearly.

Transcortical Aphasias

Transcortical aphasias are caused by damage to the watershed area which results in the loss of communication between the language areas of the brain and the rest of the cortex. The watershed area surrounds the *perisylvian zone*, the region of the brain that controls language. Because the watershed area has very few blood vessels of its own, it must get its oxygen supply from the blood that flows through it. Blood circulates quickly through the watershed area, draining into larger vessels and flowing away from the area. A TBI may result in a reduction in blood supply to the brain. Even a slight reduction can leave the watershed area without enough blood, causing trauma to the area. This damage can result in the language areas becoming isolated from the rest of the brain. When the language areas become isolated, a child may exhibit symptoms of transcortical aphasia.

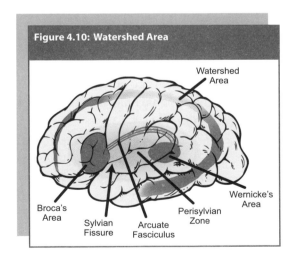

Figure 4.10: Watershed Area

Transcortical Motor Aphasia

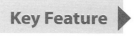 **Key Feature** ▶ problems involving the production of speech except when echoing/repeating words presented auditorily

Transcortical motor aphasia is caused by damage to the watershed area at the front of the brain around Broca's area. Clinically, transcortical motor aphasia appears very similar to Broca's-type aphasia. The one difference between the two is that the child has no difficulty repeating words he hears, and may even echo other people's speech freely (*echolalia*).

If you have a child with aphasia who appears to be Broca's-type (i.e., has dysfluent speech), ask him to repeat a series of numbers or a short phrase. If the child has no difficulty repeating the information, then a more appropriate diagnostic label would be transcortical motor aphasia.

Primary Symptoms

• symptoms are similar to Broca's-type aphasia but with good verbal repetition of auditorily presented information

Transcortical Sensory Aphasia

Key Feature ▶ problems with language comprehension, with intact ability to echo/repeat linguistic information presented auditorily

Transcortical sensory aphasia is caused by damage to the watershed area at the back of the brain around Wernicke's area. Clinically, transcortical sensory aphasia appears very similar to Wernicke's-type aphasia. The one difference between the two is that the person with transcortical sensory aphasia has no difficulty accurately repeating words he hears, and may even demonstrate echolalia.

If you have a patient with aphasia who appears to be Wernicke's-type (i.e., has deficient understanding of language), ask him to repeat a series of numbers or a short phrase. If the child has no difficulty repeating the information, then a more appropriate diagnostic label would be transcortical sensory aphasia.

Primary Symptoms

• symptoms are similar to Wernicke's-type aphasia but with good verbal repetition of auditorily presented information

Mixed Transcortical Aphasia

Key Feature ▶ problems involving the understanding of language and the production of speech except when echoing/repeating words presented auditorily

When the language areas close to the sylvian fissue (perisylvian) become isolated from the rest of the brain due to a complete watershed injury, the person can have a disorder called *mixed transcortical aphasia*. Mixed transcortical aphasia is similar to global aphasia but with one main difference—children with mixed transcortical aphasia are able to echo or repeat linguistic information they hear. The repetitions of a child with severe bilateral damage may have marked palilalia. *Palilalia* is a condition that involves abnormal repetition of syllables, words, or sometimes phrases/sentences with increasing rapidity and decreasing clarity and amplitude.

Primary Symptoms
- symptoms are similar to global aphasia but with good verbal repetition of auditorily presented information

Case Example 10 *Brian*

Brian, a four-year-old near-drowning victim, suffered a severe brain injury (*hypoxia*). The primary injury to his brain involved the watershed area.

When Brian woke up in the hospital, he was unable to understand anything that was said to him. He also could not speak spontaneously to respond to questions or to communicate his needs or wants. When Dr. Asbell spoke to him, Brian echoed her (e.g., When Dr. Asbell said, "How are you?" Brian responded, "How are you?"). Brian mimicked the words he heard with the same intonation as Dr. Asbell, but he had no comprehension of the words he was hearing and repeating. In regard to spontaneous speech, he appeared mute.

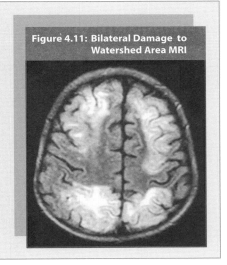
Figure 4.11: Bilateral Damage to Watershed Area MRI

General Comments Regarding Aphasia Syndromes

It is very rare to have a particular type of aphasia without difficulties that can be associated with other aphasias or cognitive disorders. Sometimes damage to selective areas of the brain can produce specific aphasias, such as Broca's-type, without other language-based problems. Usually, however, a child will have one main type of aphasia, but will show subtle signs of other types because his injury extends across different cortical regions.

As swelling and other processes of recovery resolve, the type and severity of a language disorder may change. For example, a child may begin by exhibiting global aphasia due to diffuse swelling of the brain. As the brain swelling resolves, the child may begin to show primary language deficits involving speech production rather than in understanding language. Eventually the child's primary symptoms may transition from a global aphasia to a Broca's-type aphasia. With time and recovery, the child's condition may continue to improve and be more consistent with a mild dysnomia due to ongoing word-finding difficulties. (See Appendix 4C, page 87, for a comparison of aphasia syndromes.)

As a rule, children and adolescents with TBI-related aphasias almost universally recover some language. If the damage is extensive and severe, language recovery may be limited to a few words or phrases but may be enough to allow for functional verbal communication.

When diagnosing an aphasia syndrome, describe the child's symptoms and speech-language characteristics in addition to diagnosing a specific aphasia syndrome. For example, you may diagnose a child with "global aphasia, receptive language worse than expressive," or "Wernicke's-type aphasia with dysarthria."

There are many types of problems that result from damage to the language areas of the brain. You may come across the following terms when working with children with TBI. (Note: This list is not comprehensive but covers the main syndromes.)

agraphia	a disorder of writing
alexia	a loss of previously-acquired reading skills
anomia	word-finding difficulty (i.e., know object but can't think of word)
apraxia	a disorder of learned movements that is not caused by paralysis, weakness, or incoordination, and cannot be accounted for by sensory loss. Basically, apraxia is a disorder of motor sequencing.
ataxia	muscle coordination problems most often due to cerebellar (or pathway) damage
ataxic dysarthria	coordination problems in articulation (fluctuations in articulation)
Broca's-type aphasia	a problem with the spontaneous output of speech; also called *motor, expressive,* or *dysfluent aphasia*
conduction aphasia	a problem with repetition of information
dysarthria	neuromotor difficulty in articulation and voicing
dysphagia	neuromotor difficulty in swallowing
dysphonia	neuromotor difficulty producing voice (vocal cord vibration)
echolalia	echoing (pathological repeating) words or phrases heard
global aphasia	deficits involving both receptive and expressive language
literal paraphasia	substitutions of phonemes or syllables within a word (e.g., *cabera* for *camera*); also called a *phonological* or *phomemic paraphasia*
logorrhea	excessive speech output; may be faster than normal
neologism	an expression that sounds like a word but is not an actual word (a made-up word)
palilalia	a disruption of speech fluency in which there is abnormal repetition of syllables, words, or sometimes phrases/sentences with increasing rapidity and decreasing clarity and amplitude
paraphasias	errors in speech
pure word deafness	problems with comprehension of verbal language without difficulty identifying non-linguistic sounds or with speaking, reading, or writing
telegraphic speech	speech contains mostly content words, and is often halting and dysfluent
transcortical mixed aphasia	similar to global aphasias but with intact repetition/echolalia
transcortical motor aphasia	similar to Broca's-type aphasia but with intact repetition/echolalia
transcortical sensory aphasia	similar to Wernicke's-type aphasia but with intact repetition/echolalia
verbal paraphasia	an incorrect expression of a word (e.g., calling a toothbrush a pencil)
Wernicke's-type aphasia	a problem with the extraction of the semantics (meaning) of language; can affect both receptive and expressive language; also called *fluent* or *sensory aphasia*

Area	Primary Language Function
angular gyrus (parietal lobe)	integrates language information from visual, auditory, and sensory cortex and symbolic integration for writing
arcuate fasciculus (parietal to frontal)	transmits information between Wernicke's and Broca's areas
basal ganglia/cerebellum	motor modulation/coordination for phonation and articulation
brain stem	cranial nerves responsible for oral-motor functioning and voicing
Broca's area (frontal lobe)	motor output for speech
corpus callosum	transmission of information between the two hemispheres
frontal cortex	social-pragmatics and interpersonal communication
motor cortex (frontal lobe)	articulation and oral-motor functioning
supramarginal gyrus (parietal lobe)	symbolic integration of language information for writing
thalamus	relays language information between cortical structures, naming ability, and integration with memory
watershed area	cortical area which surrounds the regions used for language
Wernicke's area (temporal/parietal region)	understanding/comprehension and encoding of language

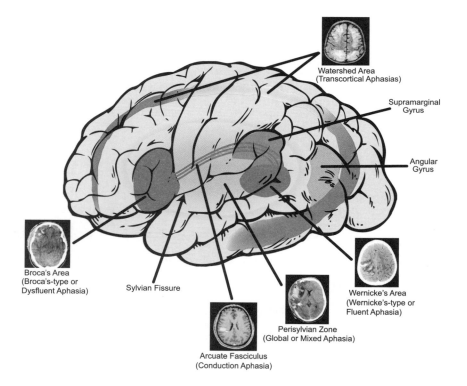

Watershed Area
(Transcortical Aphasias)

Supramarginal
Gyrus

Angular
Gyrus

Broca's Area
(Broca's-type or
Dysfluent Aphasia)

Sylvian Fissure

Arcuate Fasciculus
(Conduction Aphasia)

Perisylvian Zone
(Global or Mixed Aphasia)

Wernicke's Area
(Wernicke's-type or
Fluent Aphasia)

Nonfluent Aphasias

	Comprehension	Verbal Expression	Repetition Ability	Other Names
Broca's-type	no deficit	dysfluent, halting, effortful; may contain only meaningful words	disrupted and lacks appropriate grammar	Dysfluent, Motor, Expressive
Global	moderate to severe deficit with comprehension	dysfluent, halting, effortful, may contain only meaningful words	disrupted and lacks appropriate grammar	Mixed Aphasia
Anomic	no deficit	mostly intact fluency but pauses due to word-finding difficulty	no deficit when repeating strings of words, numbers, or letters	Anomia, Dysnomia
Transcortical Motor	no deficit	dysfluent, halting, effortful; may contain only meaningful words	no deficit when repeating strings of words, numbers, or letters	

Fluent Aphasias

	Comprehension	Verbal Expression	Repetition	Other Names
Wernicke's-type	moderate to severe deficit	fluent with many paraphasic errors; neologisms with jargon; intact syntax	disrupted and lacks appropriate grammar	Fluent, Sensory, Receptive
Conduction	no deficit	fluent but paraphasic, with pauses for word finding; poor prosody	moderate to severe deficit	
Transcortical Sensory	moderate to severe deficit	fluent with many paraphasic errors; neologisms with jargon; intact syntax	no deficit when repeating strings of words, numbers, or letters	

Chapter 5

TBI-Related Frontal Lobe Disorders

The frontal lobes are responsible for a number of higher-order functions, including executive functioning; emotional, behavioral, and social control and regulation; motor functioning; and the appropriate use of language, social pragmatics, and the subtleties of communication (e.g., understanding jokes or innuendos). Because the frontal lobes are extremely susceptible to injury due to their prominent location in the anterior section of the brain, a TBI will almost universally affect some aspect of frontal lobe functioning. This chapter discusses a variety of disorders related to frontal lobe injury as well as the cognitive effects that can result from the damage.

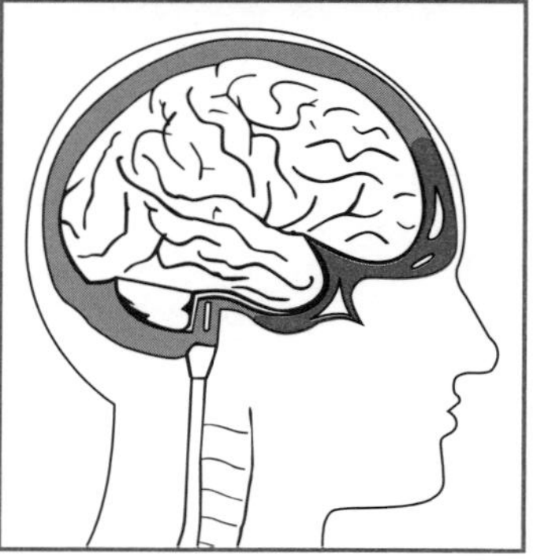

Traumatic brain injuries often result in damage to the frontal lobes. Blows to the head cause the brain to bounce off the bony structures that surround the frontal lobes, causing bruising and bleeding. Frequently, the front of a temporal lobe sustains injury at the same time. Problems resulting from this additional temporal lobe damage (e.g., memory deficits) often compound the cognitive difficulties related to the frontal lobe injury.

Figure 5.1: Bone Around Frontal and Temporal Areas

Although children with milder brain injuries, such as concussions or post-concussive syndromes, can show signs of frontal lobe dysfunction, the risk for frontal lobe dysfunction is most likely in children with moderate to severe brain injuries. Damage to the frontal lobes can cause a wide variety of symptoms, such as motor impairment, halting or disorganized speech, or even a change in a child's personality. Children may present with aphasia or verbal apraxia and/or may have trouble controlling their emotions or behavior. If the injury is close to the outside of the frontal lobe (lateral convexity), children may become passive and lack the internal drive or motivation to do the things they used to do. This was the case with Marina.

Case Example 1 *Marina*

Marina, a 14-year-old, sustained damage to both frontal lobes from a skiing accident, but she demonstrated remarkable recovery of basic cognitive skills. She achieved IQ scores within the normal range because she could rely on her prior knowledge to answer questions and complete formal evaluation tasks.

Even with intact intellectual abilities, Marina had great difficulty with everyday activities and needed supervision for most daily tasks. For example, she was unable to dress herself without help from others. She would sit on her bed without doing anything until someone told her what to do. Marina had not forgotten how to get dressed nor was she being defiant. The part of her brain that initiates activity was damaged, leaving her without self-motivation.

Executive Functioning

Executive functioning relates to one's ability to use cognitive skills efficiently in a complex environment. Executive functioning does not give us the ability to perform discrete skills, such as talk, move, or see. Instead, executive functioning regulates how we express such abilities so that we can achieve goals and function in a complex environment.

Executive functioning skills help children perform in a variety of environments smoothly, efficiently, and effectively. Even though they do not realize it, individuals rely on executive skills to get through each day. For example, adolescents who attend high school are expected to get themselves out of bed in the morning, utilize organizational and planning skills to get from class to class on time with the appropriate materials, be self-motivated to attend extra-curricular activities, allocate attentional resources despite classroom distractions, and demonstrate emotional control and appropriate social behavior during peer interactions.

Executive functions include, but are not restricted to the items in the following list. Note that the items are age-dependent—some relate to children while others relate to adolescents. For example, most young children are aware of their own abilities, older children demonstrate self-drive and self motivation, and adolescents should be using hindsight and foresight in their decision-making and problem solving.

* self-awareness of cognitive, behavioral, and physical status
* initiation of activities or internal drive
* appropriate distribution of attention and cognitive resources/energy
* higher-order problem solving and generation of strategies for success
* cognitive flexibility
* abstract reasoning
* judgment and decision making
* conceptualization of information
* creativity/originality
* maintenance of mental set and adaptation or change of mental set
* monitoring of self, others, and environmental demands/contexts/situations/social situations
* error detection and self-correction
* modification of plan, strategy, behavior
* inhibition of impulsive behaviors or thoughts
* inhibition of non-functional behaviors, such as *stereotypies* (frequent repetition of same posture, movement, or form of speech)
* organization and planning
* utilization of hindsight and feedback in addition to foresight and expectations
* volitional functioning and self-drive, self-motivation, self-initiation, and goal-directed behavior
* hypothesis testing and adaptation in addition to rule-governed behavior

Executive Dysfunction Deficits

Disrupted executive functioning, or *executive dysfunction*, results in a variety of problems. Children may retain specific cognitive abilities but have impaired ability to use such skills when necessary or appropriate. For example, a child who has executive dysfunction may have the skills and information to name as many animals as he can in one minute, but he may not be able to name any animals that begin with the letter *h* because this task requires him to organize information in a specific way.

Children and adolescents with executive dysfunction may exhibit the following functional deficits.

Organization and Planning

A child may have problems with organization, planning ahead, and noticing his mistakes. He may begin a complex task before thinking about all of the steps required to complete it. For example, if we ask him to draw a complex figure he may start drawing it too big to fit on his paper. In addition, the child may be unaware of his mistake. If we point out that he is making the figure too large, he may continue to work on his drawing without correcting the mistake.

Perseveration

Perseveration is an involuntary repetition of a thought, a behavior, an action, or a verbal utterance that continues even when it is no longer appropriate to the task at hand. For example, a child with perseveration may respond to a question correctly but then continue to repeat the same response when given new questions. He may continue to use a strategy that was appropriate for one problem on subsequent problems even though it does not work or even after he is told to change his approach.

Perseveration is frequently observed in children with executive dysfunction following a TBI. Sometimes the perseveration is mild and is exhibited only when a child is struggling to solve a complex task. At other times, the perseveration is so evident that the child is unable to do simple tasks because he gets stuck on a particular step.

The frontal lobes of the brain help people know when to move from one task or thought to another. The ability to move efficiently from task to task or from thought to thought is important when functioning in a complex, rapidly-changing environment. When a child with perseveration is in a situation in which rapid changes in thought or behavior are needed, perseveration can make it difficult for him to function.

The following are some examples of perseveration.

- We asked an adolescent to find a blank videotape in a department store and prompted him to think about where the item should be. Even though we prompted him, he got stuck on the same thought and perseverated by repeatedly going to the clothing area of the store instead of the electronics department. Once in the electronics department, he continued to look at the same items in one spot on the shelf rather than scanning across the shelves and down the aisle.

- Dr. Asbell drew one circle with the instruction to fill in the features of a clock. The child perseverated by drawing the other circles instead of filling in the clock face.

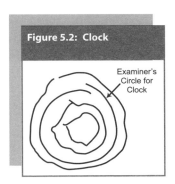

Figure 5.2: Clock

Examiner's Circle for Clock

- Dr. Lebby asked a patient with frontal injury to play Tic-Tac-Toe. Dr. Lebby drew an X in one of the empty cells. When it was the child's turn, he perseverated by drawing an X in each of the other cells.

Abstract Thinking

Children with executive dysfunction tend to think about features instead of groups or categories. For example, if you ask a child about a car, he may say that it has wheels instead of saying it is a vehicle. If you ask him in what way a dog and a cat are alike, he may say that a dog barks and a cat meows, instead of saying they are both animals.

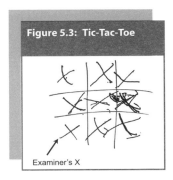

Figure 5.3: Tic-Tac-Toe

Examiner's X

Multitasking

Multitasking, or focusing on more than one thing at a time, is very difficult for children with executive dysfunction disorders. Often they can do one thing at a time as long as it is not too difficult (e.g., connect a dot-to-dot picture), but if you ask them to process multiple things at once or to alternate between two or more tasks, they may find it too difficult.

Case Example 2 *Gavin*

Gavin fell out of a second story window and sustained a large subdural hematoma when he was two years old. When Gavin was eight, his parents requested a neuropsychological evaluation because he was having learning and behavioral problems. At that time, they reported that Gavin did not seem to have any lingering problems as a result of the brain injury. During a formal examination, however, it was clear that Gavin had disrupted executive functioning skills, and they were becoming more evident as he matured.

For example, Dr. Asbell challenged Gavin with a basic task of his ability to shift focus. Gavin demonstrated little difficulty when Dr. Asbell asked him to find and cross out one object on a page. When she asked him to put an X on one object and circle another on a page, however, Gavin demonstrated multiple errors and complained, "I can't. This is way too hard." He then lost emotional control and was unable to complete the task.

Attention Difficulties

Children with executive dysfunction are often easily distracted, have poor attention to details, fail to focus on important information required to complete a task, and have problems with selective attention. Selective attention requires a child to attend to a specific stimulus feature while filtering out or ignoring others, which is difficult for a child with executive dysfunction. For example, if you ask the child to choose a specific object from several choices, he may have trouble identifying it because he over-focuses on another object that is more interesting to him.

Note: Attention difficulties may be more problematic in less-structured environments.

Judgment and Reasoning

The ability to make good decisions or to demonstrate good judgment depends on how well an individual weighs various options, given knowledge of past and current information. Following a TBI, children and adolescents often have impaired judgment and reasoning skills. They may not reason adequately to develop an appropriate course of action in a particular situation.

There are two types of reasoning skills—deductive and inductive.

1. *Deductive reasoning* is the process of making a conclusion based on previously known facts (e.g., a child must determine the card attributes you used to sort a deck of cards into two groups).

2. *Inductive reasoning* is the process of determining how to achieve a specific goal or to solve a problem (e.g., a child must determine which card attributes he will use to sort the cards into two groups).

Children and adolescents with a traumatic brain injury frequently exhibit deficits in both deductive and inductive reasoning, making it difficult for them to solve everyday problems, recognize solutions spontaneously, and consider alternate options.

Case Example 3 *Bryce*

Bryce, a 16-year-old, had bilateral frontal lobe damage due to a fall from a horse. Bryce had generally intact intelligence following his injury. His speech was a little dysarthric but intelligible, and his memory was good for day-to-day events but poor for unstructured information, such as lists of words. The most remarkable feature of Bryce's condition was his severe deficit involving executive functioning.

Bryce, continued

- He was unable to sequence normal, everyday events, such as those required for basic hygiene care or the preparation of a meal. After his accident, Bryce had to rely on cues and guidance from an occupational therapist to complete his activities of daily living.

- He had no drive or self-motivation.

- His attention was poor.

- He could not self-monitor and he had memory difficulties. When we pointed out a mistake, he seemed surprised and would correct it, but he would make a similar mistake on the next task and would again fail to recognize his error.

- Because he was unable to think about or process more than one thing at a time, Bryce lost the ability to follow multi-part directions. When we asked him to read directions one at a time, he had no difficulty reading the words; however, when we gave him all of the directions together, he was unable to sequence the steps and became confused or overwhelmed by the added complexity. Bryce also had difficulty focusing his attention on only one direction due to the visual distraction of the others. He also repeated tasks that were related to previous directions (perseveration); and due to his rigid thought processes, he mistakenly added his own rules for tasks.

Bryce's difficulties were not related to any problem he was having with language processing or intelligence. Because of his executive dysfunction, Bryce was unable to use his knowledge and skills to function independently. His organizational abilities, planning and sequencing abilities, and problem-solving skills had decreased.

Figure 5.4: Bi-Frontal Damage Around Bone

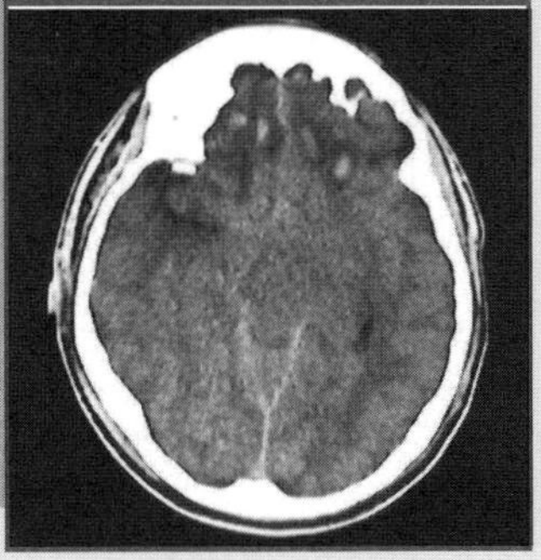

Note the damage to the frontal brain tissue close to the bones of the skull. The white is bone, the small white patches in the brain are blood, and the darker areas of brain are bruises.

Hospital Accommodations for Children with Executive Dysfunction

The external structure and accommodations provided by the staff at hospitals and clinics may make a child with executive dysfunction appear more functional than he actually is. Every day a child will get up at the same time, follow a hygiene and dressing schedule, go to therapies at the same time with the same therapists, and follow cues from the staff. All of these accommodations can lead the child's family to believe that he has no difficulties; however, when the child is discharged from the hospital his deficits may become more apparent. Therefore, while the child is still an inpatient, it is often necessary to remove him from the structured setting of the hospital in order to show his parents the difficulties he may have when he goes home, or back to school.

Case Example 4 *Amanda*

Amanda, a 13-year-old, had recovered so well after her accident that her parents believed she was "back to her pre-injury levels." Her parents, however, had only seen Amanda in the structured setting of the inpatient unit or during her therapies. Amanda's executive deficits became obvious when we asked her to find her way from our office to her room.

Amanda's room was less than 100 yards from our office with only one turn. When Amanda left our office, she turned the wrong way and walked away from her room and out of the rehabilitation unit. We walked behind her so she could not pick up cues from our behavior.

After walking to the other end of the hospital (more than 1,000 yards), we asked Amanda where she was going. She said, "Back to my room." We asked her how far her room was from our office and she replied, "Not very far." We asked, "How far have we gone since leaving the office?" She answered, "A long way." Then we asked, "So where is your room?" She looked around, spotted a nurses' station, and said, "Close to the nurses' station." Amanda looked around the nurses' station, but she did not see anything familiar and she became confused. She had not considered that there are many nurses' stations in a hospital and that this station might not be the one near her room.

We encouraged Amanda to look for signs or hospital landmarks to help her find her way back to her room. We even began to cue her to use the signs, but she became distracted by irrelevant details and was unable to focus on the important information. In the end, Amanda was unable to figure out the direction back to the rehabilitation unit, let alone to her room.

Amanda had a normal IQ and performed well in a structured setting; however, when she was removed from that setting and when supervision was taken away, her performance declined dramatically.

We see problems similar to Amanda's when patients are taken out of the inpatient or rehabilitation unit for a field trip (i.e., to a shopping mall). These field trips help identify and solve problems the children may have outside of the hospital before they are discharged.

School Accommodations for Children with Executive Dysfunction

Case Example 5 *Francis*

Francis, a 13-year-old, suffered a diffuse TBI when he crashed while riding his bicycle. Six months after his injury, Francis had returned to a regular school program. He had a tendency, however, to exhibit immature behaviors and frequently be off-task in unstructured environments. Francis's teachers reported that he "goofed off" a lot in the classroom.

We found that Francis's behavior problems in the classroom increased when he did not understand what he was supposed to be doing and when the teacher was lecturing to the class. His behavior improved when the teacher provided structure, simple directions, and cues to help him know what to do on a task.

As Francis's story illustrates, children and adolescents with TBI may have intact intellect, but they may not be able to succeed because of their executive dysfunction.

The following accommodations are very helpful in facilitating a child's performance when problems with executive functioning make it difficult for the child to function at school.

- Make the environment as consistent and as structured as possible. Children with executive dysfunction perform best in highly-structured environments. Give clear task directions and provide outlines and finished examples to help them plan and organize projects.

- Arrange tasks so they require few directions and rely on previously-learned skills. Tasks that require repetition of the same skills are easier for children with executive dysfunction because they have difficulty switching from one task to another.

- Organize work assignments so that a child does not have to think about multiple things at once.

- Teach the child to break down complex tasks into smaller units that can be done one at a time. To help the child keep track of his progress, write down the steps in order and have the child check off each step as he completes it.

- Provide cues and prompts when the child has difficulty performing a complex task.

- Help the child check his work. Point out mistakes while you help the child correct his errors. This teaches the child to check his work for mistakes, independently solve complex problems, and modify his work as necessary.

- Help the child generate novel strategies to achieve a goal. Ask the child questions, such as *How can you make a _____?* or *What will you have to do next to make _____?* Guide the child toward understanding that there are often several different ways to achieve a goal.

Affect and Emotion

Following TBI, there is often a disruption of a child's ability to control his affect and emotions. Brain-related problems involving affect and emotion can be simple or complex.

Affect

Affect is a term used to describe a child's externally displayed mood. After a TBI, the child's affect may not match his emotional status. It is very common for a child to present with a *flat affect* (lack of nonverbal or behavioral response) even though his emotional state may differ. For example, a child may have blunted or flat affect but not be sad emotionally. Similarly, a child may display an affect to suggest happiness or euphoria but in reality be depressed.

Emotion

Emotion relates to how a child feels internally. His outward presentation may or may not reflect the child's internal status. After a TBI, children may experience emotional states that are unusual for them. A child may be happy and unconcerned about his severe deficits, or he may be very depressed even while making gains in recovery.

The child's emotional state may be out of proportion to the situation or may be the opposite of what you expect. For example, children with TBI may become upset over small things and exhibit outbursts of anger. It is important to assess a child's emotional state independent of his situation. Do not assume that a child feels good because things are going well for him or that he feels depressed because things are going badly.

Irritability

Irritability and a low tolerance for frustration are common after a TBI. Irritability is usually worse soon after an injury and during the initial stages of recovery. Patients may become frustrated and lose their temper. Often their outbursts are out of proportion to the situation or the precipitating factor. Problems with irritability can last months or even years following a brain injury.

Agitation

After a TBI, many children and adolescents exhibit increased levels of agitation. This can result in outbursts of anger and expressions of profanity. Agitation after a TBI is most common within the first few days after a child's injury or after a child wakes from a coma. Usually increased states of agitation last no longer than a week; however, if there are medical complications, such as ongoing pain, disorientation, or use of restraints, increased agitation can last several weeks.

Behavior Regulation and Social Conduct

In addition to experiencing problems with affect and emotion, children with frontal lobe injuries may exhibit difficulty regulating their behavior and have problems relating to others in social contexts. These children often experience problems interpreting social pragmatics and subtleties in communication.

Behavior Regulation

During the acute stage (i.e., the first few days after an injury) following a TBI or immediately after waking from a coma, a child may exhibit excessive restlessness. Children who are restless often roll from side-to-side or attempt to stand up even if they are unable to do so due to physical injuries. Use of restraints can make the child even more restless and one-on-one supervision is often necessary to prevent the child from hurting himself.

After the acute stage, restlessness often subsides and the child may exhibit a lack of drive or motivation. The TBI may cause excessive apathy (indifference) and a lack of self-directed or goal-oriented behaviors. Apathy is most common when the damage involves the outside edges of the frontal lobes (lateral frontal cortex). Most children experience problems with motivation and apathy, while a few become disinhibited.

Case Example 6 *Ambros*

Ambros, a 17-year-old, sustained severe TBI to both of his frontal lobes. Apathy and loss of spontaneity were evident in the following short conversation he had with Dr. Asbell.

Examiner: "What do you like to do?"
Ambros: "Watch TV."

Examiner: "What do you like to watch?"
Ambros: "Nothing."

Examiner: "Do you have a favorite show?"
Ambros: "Yes."

Examiner: "What is your favorite show?"
Ambros: "Sports."

Examiner: "What is your favorite sport to watch?"
Ambros: "Soccer."

Examiner: "What else do you like to do?"
Ambros: "Hang out."

A child who is disinhibited shows a lack of behavioral control and modulation. He may say things that are socially inappropriate, may lose his temper quickly, or may have difficulty inhibiting impulsive behaviors. Disinhibition is most common when the damage involves the underside (orbital) and medial areas of the frontal lobes.

Social Conduct

The frontal lobes exert control over the parts of the brain responsible for socially-appropriate behaviors and awareness. Children with frontal lobe damage can exhibit socially-inappropriate behavior, such as saying rude or insulting things to others or acting in ways that are not appropriate to the setting or situation. We have had patients with frontal lobe injuries who have shouted obscenities and racial slurs, tried to touch or kiss others inappropriately, or said things that they would not have typically expressed.

Children with frontal lobe injuries may fail to respond to nonverbal cues given by others. These cues would normally indicate that something is unsuitable or offensive. These children also have difficulty recognizing when their behavior has made someone uncomfortable.

These behaviors can be embarrassing to the child's parents and insulting to those interacting with the child. Parents generally feel responsible for the child's behavior and may take it as a reflection on their parenting skills. Those interacting with the child may take the comments personally and become upset. If a child with frontal damage says something inappropriate to you, do not take it personally. Simply tell the child that what he said was inappropriate, give him an alternative way to express himself, and continue with the task you are working on.

Often parents and teachers do not give enough responsibility to a child who has a TBI. Even years after an injury, a child's inappropriate behaviors may be excused by parents and teachers because "he had a brain injury." Dr. Lebby's first rule of behavioral therapy for a child with a TBI is:

> ■ *A brain injury may explain bad behavior but it should not be used to excuse bad behavior. Consequences, both positive for good behavior and negative for bad behavior, are still important when working with a child who has a brain injury.* ■

Self-Centeredness

Some children with TBI have a tendency to be demanding, attention-seeking, and sometimes manipulative. They may be insensitive to the feelings or emotions of others, as well as fail to consider other people's points of view.

Case Example 7 *Ryan*

Ryan, an 11-year-old, sustained a severe diffuse TBI with significant damage to his frontal lobe when he was ejected from a motor vehicle. During the course of his hospitalization, Ryan was frequently defiant and demonstrated oppositional tendencies. Although consequences were implemented to discourage such behavior, Ryan hoarded things and often claimed that things that did not belong to him were his (e.g., therapy materials or toys that belonged to other children). This behavior indicated that Ryan would have a tendency to steal impulsively after being discharged from the hospital.

Lack of Insight

Lack of insight regarding behavioral deficits and self-awareness is common following TBI. Children fail to recognize how impulsive, irritable, childish, or demanding they are in certain situations. This lack of awareness and self-monitoring creates difficulties with interpersonal relationships when the child returns to school.

Social Communication

Children with TBI are often unable to relate well socially. They are at greater risk for being victimized due to their inability to understand when others are making fun of them, bullying them, or taking advantage of them. It is also common for children with frontal lobe dysfunction to not recognize when others are suggesting they do something inappropriate and/or dangerous. Lack of insight, disinhibition, and impulsivity also contribute to the child being gullible and/or placing himself in potentially dangerous situations.

Case Example 8 *Pilar*

When Pilar was seven years old, she sustained a head injury in a motor vehicle accident and was hospitalized for several months. When Pilar was eleven, her friends suggested that she stand on an office chair while they spun her around. Pilar, who was both energetic and impulsive, agreed. The end result was that Pilar fell off the chair, suffering a concussion.

Pilar's story is indicative of the gullibility of a young child after a TBI. We have heard numerous stories of previously brain-injured pre-teens and adolescents giving in to peer pressure and engaging in far riskier behaviors, such as drinking, driving while intoxicated, taking drugs, and becoming sexually active.

Although damage to the frontal lobes can result in motor paralysis, visual processing deficits, and problems with learning and memory, we consider these deficits to be different than those typically considered as being related to frontal lobe damage. Accordingly, motor, visual, and amnestic conditions are discussed in Chapter 6.

TBI-Related Motor, Visual, and Learning and Memory Disorders

Damage to the frontal lobes can result in motor paralyses, visual processing deficits, and problems with learning and memory; however, these conditions typically are not considered frontal lobe disorders. TBI-related motor disorders result from damage to the motor cortex, motor pathways, or deeper nuclei collectively referred to as the *basal ganglia*. Visual disorders result from damage to the visual pathways or occipital lobes (*visual cortex*). Learning and memory disorders are most often caused by bilateral damage to the hippocampi or by extensive, diffuse damage to the cortex.

Motor Disorders

There are two primary motor systems in the brain—the pyramidal system and the extrapyramidal system. The neurons from the motor cortex that send information to the spinal cord and muscles make up the *pyramidal motor system*. This system allows for voluntary control of muscles. The other parts of the brain that help control motor functioning are considered part of the *extrapyramidal motor system*. The extrapyramidal motor system helps to make muscle movements smooth and coordinated.

Pyramidal Motor System

Axons transmit information from the motor cortex to the spinal cord. Neurons in the spinal cord then relay these messages through the communication pathways to the muscles. Approximately 80 percent of the communication pathways cross over to the opposite side of the body, which means the information sent from the left side of the motor cortex controls the voluntary muscle movements on the right side of the body and vice versa. When there is an injury to one side of the motor cortex, the muscles on the opposite side of the body will be affected.

Approximately 20 percent of neurons do not cross over to the opposite side of the body. This allows for some recovery of the large muscle groups on the paralyzed side of the body (i.e., those close to the body, such as the hip, thigh, shoulder, and upper arm muscles). Smaller muscle groups (i.e., those in the wrist and the hand) receive predominately contralateral (crossed) signals. There is less chance that fine-motor dexterity will return to functional levels.

Every part of the body correlates to a specific area of the motor cortex that controls its movement. Therefore, damage to a specific area of the motor cortex will result in motor deficits to the corresponding body part. Damage to the lowest part of the motor cortex affects facial muscles and frequently speech production. It may also cause Broca's-type aphasia because Broca's area is close to the facial area of the motor cortex.

Damage to the middle of the motor cortex affects the arms and the torso, and damage to the top of the motor cortex affects the hips and legs. An easy way to remember this is to imagine an upside-down person named HAL lying on the motor strip. **HAL** stands for **H**ead, **A**rms, and **L**egs. (See Figure 1.12, page 16, for more detailed information.)

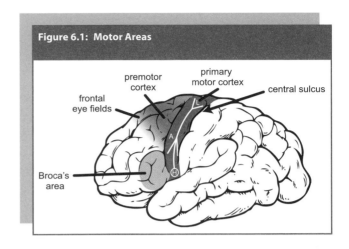

Figure 6.1: Motor Areas

Damage to the pyramidal motor system may cause minimal to severe motor weakness and will affect only the side of the body and the muscle groups that correspond to the area of injury in the motor cortex. The following conditions may result from damage to the pyramidal motor system.

- *Flaccid paralysis* is a weakness or loss of muscle tone (floppy limbs). This condition can be referred to as *hemiparesis* which is a mild to moderate degree of weakness, or as *hemiplegia* which is the severe or complete loss of motor function (paralysis).

- *Clonus* is a series of involuntary, rhythmic, muscular contractions due to a sudden, sustained muscle stretch.

- *Tremors* are rhythmic shaking movements of the limbs caused by alternating contractions of opposing muscle groups. Tremors are often present only when the child makes voluntary movements. *Intention tremors* are tremors that become worse during body movement. They usually occur during goal-directed movements and increase in severity as limb movement progresses toward the desired target.

- *Muscle atrophy* is a loss of muscle mass. Muscle atrophy is rare with damage to the brain, but it can be present if damage extends to the lower motor neurons or after the patient has been bedridden or unable to use his muscles for an extended period of time.

- *Spasticity* is increased muscle tone or resistance to passive stretching of the muscle. Immediately following an injury to the pyramidal motor system, a patient's muscles may be flaccid and floppy. The child may not be able to sustain basic body tone and posture (i.e., cannot sustain weight on his arms, legs, or trunk). Several days to weeks after the injury, there is usually a progressive increase in muscle tone as a response to passive stretching. With mild pyramidal weakness, there may be no increase in resting tone or in resistance to stretching a muscle using slow movements. With rapid stretching of the muscle, however, there may be a marked increase in tone, sometimes called a *spastic catch*. As spasticity becomes more severe, an increase in muscle resting tone may occur. Eventually, a child may develop rigidity so that it is difficult or impossible to move the limb passively.

Although spasticity is a pathological condition, there are some advantages and disadvantages to having increased tone in the limbs versus no tone (flaccid paralysis).

■ Advantages of Spasticity
  • Spasticity maintains tone in muscles that can aid in daily living activities (e.g., putting on socks/shoes).
  • Spastic tone in the legs allows a child to support his body weight and to stand and pivot when moving from place to place.
  • Muscle tone helps prevent blood from pooling in the legs. The muscles put pressure on the veins, pushing the blood out of the legs and back to the heart.

■ Disadvantages of Spasticity
  • Spasticity can interfere with performing daily living activities (e.g., if a child cannot bend his arms, putting on a shirt is difficult).
  • Increased muscle tone may mask the return of voluntary movement.
  • Severe spasticity may lead to *contractures* (permanent shortening of the muscles) or to dislocation of joints.
  • Spasticity may cause increased pain due to the tight muscles.

Extrapyramidal Motor System

The extrapyramidal motor system is important for the initiation, coordination, and guidance of voluntary movements. The primary extrapyramidal motor structures are the basal ganglia and the cerebellum. These structures make muscle movements smooth and coordinated, and they modulate the functioning of the pyramidal system.

Basal ganglia structures link automatic movements with voluntary movements to help a child adapt to environmental needs. For example, when a child picks up an object from a table, the automatic movements he requires for a normal standing posture become linked to the voluntary movements he requires to reach for and grasp the object. The basal ganglia also function to change the inhibition and excitation of different muscle processes, depending on environmental needs.

Damage to the basal ganglia can cause an inability to start or stop movements. A child with basal ganglia damage may have trouble initiating movement and may just stand in one place for a long time or sit on a bed motionless. These symptoms are similar to those seen in *Parkinson's disease* as they involve similar areas of the basal ganglia. Other children may have damage to areas of the basal ganglia similar to patients with *Huntington's disease*. These children may have trouble stopping their movements and appear to be in constant motion. Children may also produce automatic movements when they are not needed. These involuntary movements are seen in tic disorders, such as Tourette's syndrome.

Damage to the cerebellum can also cause problems with coordination of movements. A child with damage to the cerebellum exhibits motor functioning similar to a person who is intoxicated. Children with cerebellar damage have difficulty walking and making accurate movements required for processes such as dressing, writing, and drawing.

Damage to the extrapyramidal system can also cause ballism. *Ballism* is a severe form of involuntary movement disorder. It involves abnormal swinging, jerking, or shaking movements of the arms or legs, especially when the child is trying to use them to complete a motor task. Ballism is most often caused by damage to the deep nuclei of the brain.

Case Example 1 *Yvonne*

Yvonne, a two-year-old, was admitted to the hospital with an injury caused by suspected non-accidental trauma. Yvonne presented with diffuse injury to her brain. This resulted in damage to the extrapyramidal system, causing ballism. Yvonne needed to wear special padded boots to prevent her from bruising her ankles and calf muscles because the constant motion of her legs resulted in her continually kicking her wheelchair. When playing with toys, Yvonne's arms would jerk suddenly, making it extremely difficult for her to voluntarily manipulate her toys.

Damage to the extrapyramidal motor system can also result in the following conditions.

- *akinesia*—loss of, or absence of, voluntary movement

- *ataxia*—problems with coordination, usually associated with an injury to the cerebellum or cerebellar pathways

- *athestosis*—slow, writhing movements of the fingers and hands and sometimes the tongue, toes, or limbs

- *bradykinesia*—extreme slowing of body movements

- *chorea*—involuntary movements of the limbs and facial muscles. Movements can be forceful, jerky, rapid, or rhythmic

- *dyskinesia*—involuntary movements that are repetitive or stereotyped, such as shrugging the shoulders or turning the head

- *dystonia*—the sustained increase in agonist and antagonist muscles that move a joint. Because the pull is strong and often asymmetrical, the joint may take on an odd or twisted posture. Dystonia may produce a lasting change in the position of the joint (limb or trunk), or it may be a dramatic, sudden movement, often elicited by intentional movement.

- Parkinsonian-type tremors when resting that may subside with voluntary movement

Apraxia

The brain stores patterns of motor sequences so that an individual does not have to think about making complex movements. After a TBI, these motor patterns may be disrupted or lost altogether causing apraxia. *Apraxia* is a disorder of motor planning or sequencing. The child with apraxia is unable to perform everyday tasks requiring complex or skilled motor movements, such as walking, brushing teeth, tying shoelaces, and speaking.

Apraxia syndromes can affect any voluntary muscle system. The most common apraxia syndromes involve the arms, legs, and oral-motor system. The general appearance of an apraxia is when the child has the physical ability to perform the necessary individual movements required for a complex motor skill but cannot sequence the movements to complete the compound task. For example, a child may be able to move his legs and feet but may not be able to sequence the movements in order to walk. With oral-motor apraxia, the child may be able to put his tongue in the correct place during involuntary actions (e.g., smiling, licking, chewing), but may not be able to make the necessary voluntary movements or sequence his tongue movements on command to produce phonemes and words, especially those that are polysyllabic.

Unlike most brain-related syndromes, apraxia syndromes are not defined by a child's symptoms as much as they are by exclusion, the ruling out of other causes of the motor problem. Apraxia is NOT caused by:

- muscle weakness
- poor coordination
- loss of normal muscle tone or posture
- loss of sensation

- poor cooperation
- intellectual deficit
- pyramidal or extrapyramidal motor signs

Case Example 2 *Michael*

Michael, an eight-year-old, was injured during a baseball game when the bat slipped out of the batter's hands and hit Michael on the left side of his head. Michael sustained a skull fracture and severe damage to the left perisylvian region, the tissue lying under the skull fracture.

Once Michael's brain swelling resolved, he was left with a very severe oral-motor apraxia syndrome, which prevented him from speaking. He was able to produce the sounds *ooh* or *aarh*, but he could not voluntarily produce single verbal sounds, such as /ba/ or /da/. He also had to concentrate very hard in order to do simple oral-motor tasks, such as blowing or trying to make a single consonant sound.

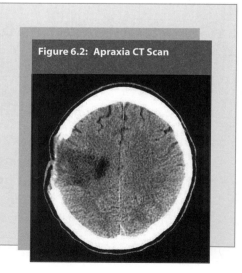

Figure 6.2: Apraxia CT Scan

Dysarthria

Dysarthria is a speech disorder that is characterized by weakness or incoordination of muscles used for speech. Dysarthria is generally caused by damage to the cerebellum, the brain stem, or the nerve fibers that connect these structures. The cerebellum, brain stem, and motor cortex control the muscles used to make sounds and/or to coordinate movements of the lips, tongue, palate, and vocal folds.

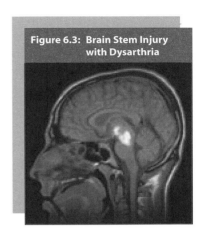

Figure 6.3: Brain Stem Injury with Dysarthria

Dysarthric speech may be slow, weak, slurred, poorly articulated, or incoordinated. It can be caused by too much or too little muscle tone in the tongue and mouth muscles or by a problem with the coordination of movement between the tongue and mouth muscles (*ataxic dysarthria*).

Visual Disorders

Disorders of the visual system can be extremely complex and may involve a number of brain regions. Visual disorders can be caused by damage to the optic nerves; the pathways to the deeper structures of the brain, specifically the lateral geniculate nuclei of the thalamus; pathways from the thalamus to the cortex; or multiple areas of visual cortex that are used to process visual information. This section will introduce some of the more common visual disorders caused by TBI and focus on conditions that most affect a child's functioning. (See Appendix 6A on page 115 for a summary of visual disorders caused by brain injury.)

Visual Processing by the Primary Visual Cortex

Visual information travels from the eyes to the thalamus and then from the thalamus to the visual cortex (occipital lobe). The visual information received by the cortex is arranged using the same organization as images on the retina (*retinotopic*). For example, if the image projected to the retina is a dog near a tree, the same organization of items will be retained throughout the visual pathways and all the way to the cortex.

A *visual field* is the entire area of the environment that the child sees when he is looking forward, including what he sees with his peripheral vision. The visual information is split into two visual fields—the *right visual field* (everything visible on the right) and the *left visual field* (everything visible on the left).

- The relationships between the visual fields and the areas of the brain that process information are as follows.
    - Information from the left visual field is sent to the right hemisphere of the brain.
    - Information from the right visual field is sent to the left hemisphere of the brain.

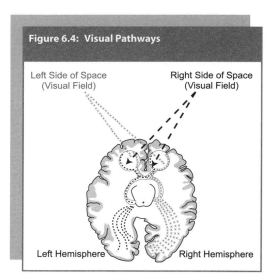

Figure 6.4: Visual Pathways

Left Side of Space (Visual Field)

Right Side of Space (Visual Field)

Left Hemisphere

Right Hemisphere

- The visual fields are also split top to bottom.
    - Information from above the point of fixation is sent to the bottom of the visual cortex.
    - Information from below the point of fixation is sent to the top of the visual cortex.

- Peripheral visual information is also processed by the visual cortex.
    - Information close to fixation is sent to the back of the visual cortex—the occipital pole at the back of the brain.
    - Information from the periphery is sent to areas deeper in the cortex—away from the occipital pole.

Damage to different parts of the visual cortex will result in disrupted vision in specific areas of visual space.

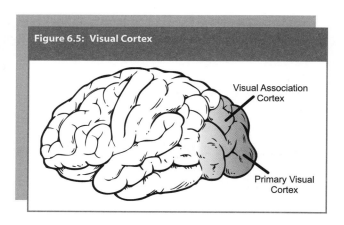

Figure 6.5: Visual Cortex

Visual Association Cortex

Primary Visual Cortex

- If a child has brain damage to the right hemisphere's visual cortex, he will be "blind" for information within the left visual field. This is known as a *left hemianopia*. Similarly, damage to the visual cortex of the left hemisphere will produce a right-sided hemianopia.

- If a child has brain damage to the upper part of the left hemisphere's visual cortex, he will have a blind area within the right visual field below fixation. This is called a *quadranopia* (loss of information in one of the four quadrants: upper right, upper left, lower right, or lower left).

- Loss of a part of the visual field that does not correspond to a half (hemianopia) or quarter (quadranopia) is called a *scotoma*.

Patients with hemianopia, quadranopia, or a scotoma may not be aware of their deficits. Those that are aware can compensate quite well by scanning a visual scene using eye and head movements.

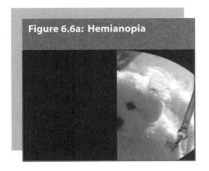

Figure 6.6a: Hemianopia

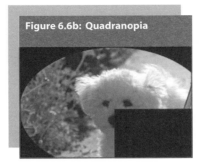

Figure 6.6b: Quadranopia

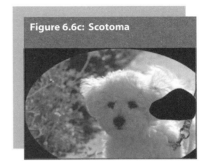

Figure 6.6c: Scotoma

Case Example 3 *Cheryl*

Cheryl, an 11-year-old, injured her left occipital lobe when she hit the back of her head during a gymnastics practice session. Her injury resulted in a right hemianopia; and she was unable to see anything presented to the right side of where she was looking. She was able to compensate by moving her eyes and head to scan the entire visual environment. This strategy allowed Cheryl to accommodate for her injury quite well. Cheryl was able to return to school and complete her work with few accommodations. Her performance improved once she got into the habit of scanning the page to see if she missed anything.

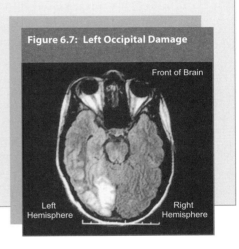

Figure 6.7: Left Occipital Damage

Front of Brain

Left Hemisphere

Right Hemisphere

Visual Processing Outside of the Primary Visual Cortex

Problems with visual processing can also be caused by damage to the areas between the primary visual cortex and the parietal or temporal lobes. As a general rule, damage to the area and pathways between the primary visual cortex and the top of the parietal lobe can disrupt awareness of object location in space (i.e., *where*). Damage to the area and pathways between the primary visual cortex and the lower part of the parietal lobe and to the temporal lobes can disrupt the ability to identify objects (i.e., *what*).

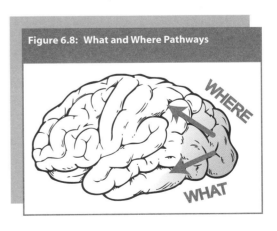

Figure 6.8: What and Where Pathways

WHERE

WHAT

Common disorders resulting from damage to the areas between the primary visual cortex and the parietal or temporal lobes include:

- *visual agnosia*—the inability to recognize objects
- *prosopagnosia*—the inability to recognize faces
- *visual neglect*—the failure to attend to stimuli in the visual field opposite from the damaged hemisphere (e.g., damage to the right hemisphere can lead to neglect on the left side of the environment, and vice versa)

The following case examples demonstrate some of the problems faced by children with visual agnosia, prosopagnosia, and visual neglect.

Visual Agnosia and Prosopagnosia

Children who have visual agnosia and prosopagnosia can see, but they are unable to recognize objects or faces. They have intact visual perception and can describe or draw objects and faces, but they don't know what the objects, faces, or pictures represent. This is a visual recognition problem, not a naming problem.

Case Example 4 *Julia*

Julia, a 16-year-old, fell and hit her head while ice-skating. Her brain injury was restricted to the right parietal region which helps to visually identify objects. The MRI scan in Figure 6.9 shows a top view of Julia's brain. The damaged area (identified by the arrow) swelled so much that it was necessary to cut her skull to relieve the pressure in her brain.

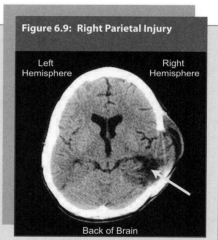

Figure 6.9: Right Parietal Injury

Left Hemisphere — Right Hemisphere

Back of Brain

The skull is white and the brain is gray. The dark, fluid-filled areas, identified by the arrow, indicate cell damage or tissue removed during surgery.

After her brain injury, Julia had visual agnosia and prosopagnosia. When Julia saw pictures of common objects, she said they looked like modern art paintings—just a series of random shapes and lines. Her ability to remember faces was also very impaired. Dr. Lebby asked Julia to study some pictures of faces. Later, he showed Julia the pictures again and asked her if she had seen them before. She performed at chance levels (50/50) and was unable to recognize even the familiar faces of her parents and friends.

Julia had a very high Verbal Intelligence Quotient (VIQ=121, 94th percentile) although her brain injury resulted in her achieving a very low Performance Intelligent Quotient (PIQ <56. <1st percentile). Even though Julia was intelligent and had excellent language skills, she was unable to make sense of things visually.

Julia's deficits included, but were not restricted to, the following difficulties.
- discriminating a toothpaste tube from shampoo
- dressing because she could not visually orient her clothing (e.g., she did not know where her arms went when looking at a shirt)

Julia, continued

- recognizing her friends
- distinguishing the television remote from the cordless phone
- understanding television shows because she could not identify people or objects
- putting away dishes because she could not determine which dish she had in her hand
- reading a clock or a speedometer
- making sense of the visual flow of traffic when riding in a car

Julia's visual deficits made it very difficult for her to function independently after her discharge from the hospital. Several years after her accident, Julia reported that her visual deficits were not as severe as they were during the first year after her injury, but they were still evident. By the time she entered college, Julia had learned to compensate for her impaired ability to recognize objects by putting labels on items and then reading the labels.

Patients with visual agnosia, like Julia, compensate by using other senses. They depend on tactile, auditory, and olfactory senses to help them identify objects. Sometimes, however, TBI can also disrupt more than one sensory modality, making object identification very difficult. For example, Julia had problems compensating for her visual disorder using touch as she also had ***astereognosis***, the loss of the ability to recognize objects by handling them.

Visual Neglect

Damage to the right side of the brain can cause left visual neglect syndrome. A child with left visual neglect syndrome will not pay attention to the left side of whatever he is looking at (e.g., the landscape, objects, himself). Damage to the left side of the brain can also produce a right-sided neglect, although it is less common.

A child with visual neglect has the ability to move his attention to the neglected area of space, but it often takes a very salient stimulus, external cueing, and a conscious effort. In other words, he lacks the ability to unconsciously and automatically focus his attention to the neglected area. When a child is not deliberately focusing on information from the neglected area, he has a strong bias to ignore that information in favor of information coming from the non-neglected part of his visual field.

Because most patients are unaware of their visual neglect syndrome, they are unable to compensate by scanning an object, scene, or page. You can help children overcome neglect by providing them with cues and reminders to move their attention to the neglected side. Although you will be able to attract a child's attention to the neglected visual field, the awareness will only last a short time. Usually, within seconds, the child will again neglect that side of space.

▶ Complex Visual Processing and Visual Neglect

Damage to areas of the brain between the visual cortex and the parietal or temporal lobes frequently results in disruption of complex visual processing and in visual neglect. The following case example demonstrates how a child can have problems with the allocation of attention to visual space and with processing complex visual information.

Case Example 5 *Miguel*

Miguel, a nine-year-old, was injured when he was hit by a car while walking his dog. His brain injury was predominantly within his left parietal lobe, resulting in a right-sided visual neglect syndrome. Miguel also had damage in his visual association cortex, close to his primary visual cortex. Because his primary visual cortex was not severely damaged, Miguel could see well enough for basic functioning. His injury, however, made it difficult for him to process visual information and make sense of the things he saw, especially things that were complex or small (e.g., a puzzle).

Miguel's teachers initially believed that his brain injury caused him to lose the ability to read and to do mathematics. We discovered that Miguel's reading and math skills were fully intact but he could not see normal-sized text because of his visual processing difficulties. By using extra-large print (i.e., over three inches in height), Miguel was able to read and do math problems at grade level.

Miguel's visual neglect syndrome made his situation even more complicated because he failed to pay attention to the information on the right side of sentences and math problems. For example, Miguel was able to solve math problems but would continually neglect the numbers on the right side. As you can see in Figure 6.11, he accurately solved the math problem if you ignore the digits on the right (the 1 and 7).

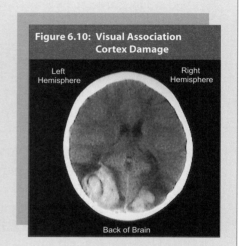

Figure 6.10: Visual Association Cortex Damage

Left Hemisphere — Right Hemisphere

Back of Brain

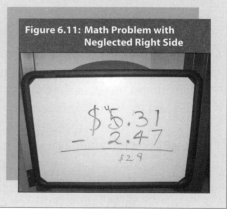

Figure 6.11: Math Problem with Neglected Right Side

Children with visual processing deficits or neglect syndromes have difficulty functioning at school. Teachers can misinterpret difficulties as being related to intelligence or achievement instead of being related to a sensory disorder involving vision or neglect. We frequently contact school teachers (with parental permission) to discuss ways to accommodate a child's difficulties.

We accommodated Miguel's deficits by using a dry-erase board and large letters, words, and numbers and cued him to look at the entire problem or sentence. At school, Miguel used a large magnifying screen to complete his work, and an aide cued Miguel to look at information on the right side of the page. These accommodations often work well for children who have visual processing deficits and/or neglect.

▶ Left Hemianopia and Left Visual Neglect

The following case example demonstrates how damage to areas of the brain involving the visual cortex and the region between the visual cortex and parietal lobes can result in a child having a combination of left hemianopia and left visual neglect.

Case Example 6 *Ian*

Ian, a 15-year-old, sustained a severe brain injury when he was hit by a car while riding a motor scooter without a helmet. His injury affected most of his right hemisphere. The damage involved many areas, including the right parietal lobe and visual cortex. Ian had both a left–sided hemianopia (blind to information on the left side) and a left visual neglect syndrome (did not pay attention to the left side of things he could see). Even though Ian could see everything around him if he moved his head, he still did not attend to some information due to his visual neglect syndrome.

Tests of neglect can be used in patients with hemianopia because neglect is a problem with the child's allocation of attention to what he sees, even when he only sees half of the visual field. To demonstrate Ian's left-sided neglect, Dr. Lebby drew the stem of a flower and a circle to represent the center of the flower. He then asked Ian to draw the petals on the flower. Ian's finished picture did not have any petals on the left side of the flower. (See Figure 6.13a.) Dr. Lebby also drew a circle and asked Ian to make a clock by adding the numbers and drawing the hands to show 9:50. Ian's attempt is shown in Figure 6.13b.

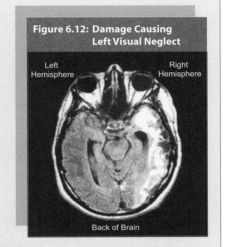

Figure 6.12: Damage Causing Left Visual Neglect

Left Hemisphere · Right Hemisphere

Back of Brain

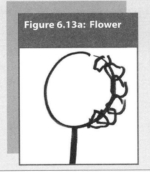

Figure 6.13a: Flower

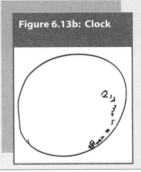

Figure 6.13b: Clock

Amnestic Syndromes (Learning and Memory)

A TBI can leave previous memories predominantly intact, while affecting the ability to store and/or retrieve new memories and to learn new information. Memory-based deficits after a brain injury range from mild difficulty with new learning, to the inability to recall information from only a few seconds earlier. Impaired memory for events that took place before the injury can also be caused by a TBI. Memory disorders can be categorized into two primary types—anterograde amnesia and retrograde amnesia.

1. *anterograde amnesia*—the loss of the ability to learn and remember new information after an injury

2. *retrograde amnesia*—the loss of memories stored before the injury

> Impaired attentional functioning is one of the most common reasons a child has difficulty with learning and memory following a TBI. When a child does not pay attention to the information being presented, he cannot store it in his memory.

A TBI that causes anterograde amnesia affects a child's ability to consolidate new information and integrate it with past knowledge, making it difficult for him to remember things. Many times, however, the child's memory functioning is not the primary problem. A TBI can also disrupt the various processes and cognitive skills needed for efficient learning, resulting in learning and memory difficulties. For example, a child with language impairments will have difficulty learning and remembering information presented verbally, and a child with visual impairments will have difficulty learning and remembering visual information due to his poor ability to process or understand the material. When the injury involves the temporal lobes, the deep mid-thalamic structures, or the frontal lobes, children may have amnestic syndromes that last indefinitely. The specific effects of brain damage on learning and memory depend on the brain structures that are injured.

Temporal Lobe Amnesia

Memory problems are common after a TBI because the temporal lobes are prone to damage during a closed head injury. The hippocampi are located deep and medially within the temporal lobes and are directly involved with memory functioning. The hippocampi are connected to almost every area of cortex and to almost all subcortical structures, allowing them to store new memories and retrieve old memories when needed.

Damage to the hippocampi or the pathways between the hippocampal structures and other parts of the brain will disrupt the storage of memories and new learning. Temporal lobe damage can also disrupt the retrieval of old memories, but this is not as big a problem as the storage of new memories. Often, short-term memory remains intact. The child can retain information for a few minutes using mental rehearsal techniques and contextual cues, but, as soon as he is distracted, he forgets the new information.

Children who have problems learning new information often do not have difficulty learning motor skills. If a child is doing a new task, such as tracing a design while looking in a mirror, he will improve with practice. He will not, however, remember doing the task; it will be "new" to him each time. This type of skill learning has been called *procedural memory* (i.e., non-declarative memory) because it involves the learning of motor procedures.

Children with temporal lobe amnesia also develop a familiarity with repeated exposure to the same information. For example, they may not remember being asked to memorize a short list of words but, when given choices, they may pick the words they heard previously because they sound "familiar." These children generally say that they are guessing, but their guesses can be quite accurate.

Case Example 7 *Kyle*

Kyle was 17 years old when he had a severe brain injury from a motorcycle accident. He injured both temporal lobes and much of the frontal cortex. Kyle had an extreme case of profound anterograde amnesia with mild retrograde amnesia.

Even though Dr. Lebby saw Kyle every day, Kyle never learned who Dr. Lebby was and he was always unaware that he was in the hospital. Each time, Kyle thought it was the first time he had been in the exam room and he did not know why he was there. When Dr. Lebby asked Kyle where he was, Kyle would look around and guess based on what he saw. Whenever Dr. Lebby told Kyle he had been in the hospital for several months, Kyle always responded, "Are you serious? It feels like I've only been here today."

One day, Dr. Lebby gave Kyle a story to remember and then left the exam room for exactly 60 seconds. When he returned, Kyle introduced himself as if he had never seen Dr. Lebby before, and he had no memory of the story he had just read.

Unfortunately, Kyle's memory functioning has not changed significantly since his injury. He has not retained new memories since his accident. He is now legally an adult and has no memory of aging. The last time Dr. Lebby saw him, Kyle still said he was 17. When Dr. Lebby told him he was 21, Kyle's response was, "Are you serious?"

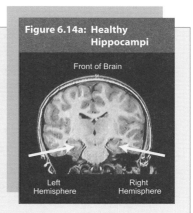

Figure 6.14a: Healthy Hippocampi

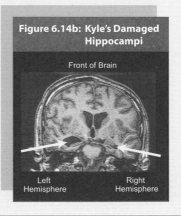

Figure 6.14b: Kyle's Damaged Hippocampi

Diencephalic Amnesia

Damage to the mid-thalamic structures within the diencephalon can result in both retrograde and anterograde memory loss. A child with diencephalic amnesia syndrome often lacks insight or awareness regarding his memory problems. He will also be disoriented for time and location; he can tell you his name, but cannot tell you the time or where he is.

Damage to the mid-thalamic structures and mammillary bodies can also cause confabulations. A *confabulation* is the production of a false memory (i.e., remembering something that did not happen because the brain fills in the missing information). Often, confabulated memories relate to actual events in the child's life or to something he has witnessed. Confabulations are often difficult to discriminate from real memories without firsthand knowledge of what actually happened.

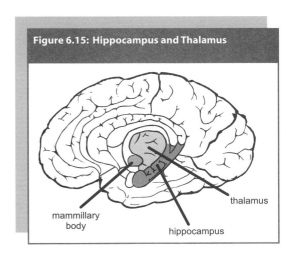

Figure 6.15: Hippocampus and Thalamus

thalamus

mammillary body

hippocampus

Confabulations are evident when you ask a child with diencephalic amnesia to recall a story that someone read to him. Although he may remember some information from the story, he will add false memories and other information to the story. The child is not guessing or making up the information. His brain makes him think that the information and the memories are real.

Case Example 8 *David*

David, a 16-year-old, was involved in a motor vehicle accident. He injured the deep midline structures of his brain, including the diencephalon and mammillary bodies. After David woke up from his coma, he was unable to store new memories, and his recollection of what happened to him changed every few minutes. For example, David watched his mother sign medical consent forms and watched a war movie with his brother. He also tried to get up from his wheelchair to "walk home," but was prevented from doing so. Later, David had no memories of these events but reported memories of things that did not happen. He said he was a soldier and received his injuries in battle. He said his mother sent him to war and he "remembered" seeing her sign his enlistment papers. He also "remembered" that Dr. Lebby was a guard at a prisoner of war camp and that he had restrained David when he tried to escape.

Confabulations elicit the same emotional responses that would be expected of true memories because patients believe they are true. David confabulated that he saw his father killed in the war. He cried uncontrollably for the loss of his father and the trauma it caused. When Dr. Lebby told David that his father was still alive and visited him every night, David said, "You're lying to me to try and make me feel better." Fortunately, after a few minutes David forgot what he was crying about and went on as if nothing had happened.

As David recovered, his ability to make sense of information improved. He began to realize that his memories were not real, and he began to recognize his confabulations. David's amnestic syndrome improved dramatically over the next three months. One year later, David's memory functioning was close to normal levels and his confabulations had ended.

Cortically-Based Amnesia

Severe diffuse damage to the frontal cortex can result in a variety of symptoms involving memory functioning, such as:

- problems storing new memories
- difficulty retrieving old memories
- poor recall of temporal order
- difficulty with *source memory* or *episodic memory* (i.e., unable to remember where the child heard something or the situation in which the child learned something)
- deficits with insight or awareness of one's memory limitations

A child with cortically-based amnesia may also experience confabulations, even though they are generally the result of damage to the diencephalic structures. Executive dysfunction, disrupted source or episodic memory, and deficient insight all contribute to a child being unable to identify, self-monitor, and/or correct false memories.

▶ **achromatopsia**
a loss of color perception which may be present in the whole visual field, half of the visual field (*hemiachromatopsia*), or a quarter of the visual field (*quadrachromatopsia*)

▶ **agnosia syndrome**
a condition in which there is a loss of recognition for visually-based information

- **letter/word agnosia**
  also called *alexia*; a specific visual disorder involving reading which causes a disruption of a child's previously-attained ability to recognize written information (i.e., letters, numbers, and/or words)

- **prosopagnosia**
  the inability to recognize faces even with intact visual processing ability, good face discrimination, intact memory functioning, and normal intellect; a specific agnosia syndrome for faces (i.e., children know that they are looking at a face but cannot recognize the person)

- **simultagnosia**
  difficulty perceiving multiple objects simultaneously from a complex scene; visual attention narrowed to a single entity and patient neglects other objects in the scene

- **visual agnosia**
  the inability to recognize an object (real or pictured) even though sensory functions are intact (good vision); can be present with intact intellect, memory, and language functioning

▶ **anopia syndrome**
a condition in which there is a loss of visual perception corresponding to the area of damage

- **Charles Bonnet syndrome**
  syndrome characterized by the presence of complex visual hallucinations that occur within the blind areas of a visual field, such as where there is a hemianopia

- **hemianopia**
  loss of visual perception to half of the visual field; damage to visual structures or pathways on one side of the brain causes loss of visual perception for information in the visual field on the opposite side (e.g., damage to right visual cortex [occipital lobe] can result in a left hemianopia)

- **quadranopia**
  loss of visual perception to a quarter of the visual field; damage to the visual structures or pathways on one side of the brain plus damage on the top or bottom of the visual cortex (e.g., damage to right visual cortex [occipital lobe] at bottom of brain can result in loss of visual perception in left upper quadrant of space)

- **scotoma**
  loss of visual perception to a region of the visual field that does not correspond to a particular hemi-field (hemianopia) or quadrant (quadranopia); can vary in shape and size and often relates to small areas of damage involving the visual pathways or visual cortex

▶ **strabismus**
a condition in which there is a misalignment of the eyes

- **diplopia**
  double vision because of lack of coordinated eye movements

- **dysconjugate gaze/tracking**
  a problem with coordinated movements of the eyes; eyes not moving together causes brain to receive visual images from each eye that are not coordinated; can be caused by disruption of nerve or muscle functions required to move either eye, often resulting in diplopia

- **esotropia**
  a condition in which an eye does not move laterally (outward) and becomes turned in toward the nose; may involve one or both eyes (cross-eyed)

- **exotropia**
  a condition in which an eye does not move medially (inward) and becomes turned out away from the nose; may involve one or both eyes

▶ **visual neglect**
a bias to unconsciously focus attention on the non-neglected area to the detriment of the neglected area; attention can be attracted to neglected area, but awareness lasts only a short time

Chapter 7

General Assessment Issues

Most people would say that a test of brain functioning evaluates cognitive or language ability; however, we believe that clinicians evaluate cognition and language functioning and utilize tests to assist them. Tests are tools that aid in the identification of specific cognitive, behavioral, or emotional strengths and weaknesses. Formal tests are necessary to compare a child's functioning with that of other children matched by age, grade, and other features, such as ethnicity. For children with a traumatic brain injury, the data from these tests is meaningless unless it is integrated with other information. It is important to integrate formal test data with clinical knowledge of the child's pre-injury development and behavior, and with your observation of the child in less-structured settings. The information provided in this chapter can be applied to a variety of clinical situations, settings, types of brain injury, and neurocognitive syndromes.

▌ Considerations for Testing

Evaluating cognitive functioning after a brain injury can be complex, even if the evaluation is restricted to a specific function, such as language. Damage to areas of the brain not specifically related to language may cause a wide variety of symptoms that can significantly influence a child's functional language. For example:

- Children with poor attention may not respond to verbal questions, may respond to only part of a question, may have difficulty when given multiple directions, or may complete only the first or last part of a multi-step direction.

- Children with short-term memory deficits may have difficulty responding to long questions or written passages. This difficulty may be due to the inability to remember all of the information and not a result of a language disorder.

- Frontal lobe injuries that result in executive dysfunction can lead to disorganized speech and language patterns.

- Fatigue can make any difficulty more apparent and frustrating for the child.

Demands for efficient processing and multitasking are different on various tests of cognition. Therefore, children with TBI may have problems with processing efficiency on some tests but not on others. For example, children with TBI score relatively well on standardized tests, such as an IQ test. An IQ test is given in a controlled environment and many of the tasks do not have strict time constraints. IQ tests also rely on prior learning and knowledge or abilities which are often retained in children with TBI. On the other hand, children with brain injuries may not perform or score well on tests that measure executive functions, such as rapid processing speed, multitasking, flexibility of problem solving, and cognitive efficiency.

Test data for children without TBI is often more straightforward and easier to interpret than test data for children with TBI. When testing a child with a brain injury, the test results can be misleading because of insufficient background data and/or the child's deficits in neurocognitive functioning. In order to successfully assess the child with TBI, it is important to implement the following strategies.

- Consider these important factors when assessing a child's brain injury and his language and cognitive skills post-injury.
  - severity of the injury
  - parts of the brain that were most injured
  - type of injury (diffuse or focal)
  - age of the child
  - the child's functioning prior to the injury
  - resources available to the child that assist in recovery and rehabilitation

- Conduct tests in the child's preferred language. If the child is bilingual, it is best to test him in both languages. Testing in different languages allows you to better understand how the child may function in different environments. For example, if a child speaks English in school and Spanish at home, his parents may not be aware of his difficulties communicating at school.

- Evaluate a child's language functioning when he is speaking with adults and when he is speaking with his peers. Children with TBI often have less difficulty communicating with adults or older children who repair conversation breakdowns and/or fill in missing information. Communication may end rapidly with peers who are not capable of interpreting the inadequacies that often occur after brain injury (e.g., word-finding problems, dysarthric speech, lack of affect).

- Use more than one test to evaluate cognitive functioning. Because children with brain injuries exhibit highly variable functioning, one test is inadequate. Use a variety of measures, making sure to include some that are highly-structured and some that are more complex with time constraints. Using a variety of tests will provide you with a better idea of the child's basic skills as well as his cognitive efficiency.

- Evaluate functioning in more than one environment when possible. Even though a child may do well in a one-on-one testing environment, he may not be able to perform in a less-structured environment or in a group situation. This is because the one-on-one environment does not have the complexities of real-world situations, and therefore, the child's executive functioning difficulties may not be apparent.

- Evaluate for strengths. Do not be so concerned with documenting deficits that you forget to highlight a child's strengths. Strengths are just as important as deficits. Describing a child's strengths allows others to use them to help the child overcome his weaknesses or deficits.

- Use normative data cautiously. Data derived from large populations may not relate to the specific child you are evaluating due to differences in the child's life experiences, such as his culture, language, and educational background.

- Consider both a child's age and his functional ability levels. An assessment based only on the child's chronological age may not be appropriate if the child functions well below age-expected levels. For example, giving a language test designed for children six years and above to a seven-year-old child with a brain injury may not be the best option. If the child functions at a two-year-old level, he would not be able to complete even the easiest items on the test. Instead, consider using a test that is designed for children who function within his ability and performance level. Although you cannot compare the child's performance to the normative data provided by the test, you can provide a descriptive evaluation of the child's ability and approximate age-equivalency.

- Take into account normal development of the brain as well as abnormal development resulting from a TBI when developing assessment techniques. Brain injury can change the normal developmental course of cognitive skills and therefore should be considered during assessment. For example, when assessing nonverbal reasoning skills in a child who had a TBI that affected language functioning, you may want to choose tests that do not use complex verbal instructions or require the child to provide lengthy verbal responses.

- Consider a child's perceptual or motor deficits. A young child may not know that something is wrong with his perceptual or motor system and may fail tests designed to measure other skills. Older children can compare their past experiences to their current functioning while younger children cannot. The following example demonstrates how a young child may not report difficulties because he does not realize his deficits are abnormal.

Case Example 1 *Max*

Max sustained a closed-head injury after falling from a playground slide when he was three years old. Over the next two years, Max tested poorly on visual tasks during his examinations. One day he asked Dr. Asbell, "Why are there two moons in the picture?" Max was seeing double. He had been seeing double since his injury, but he never complained about it because he did not know it was abnormal.

- Be aware of other reasons a child may perform or appear to perform poorly on a test that have nothing to do with a brain injury or cognitive dysfunction. These reasons include lack of effort, fatigue, poor vision, poor hearing, and emotional factors. For example, if a child is upset with his parents for bringing him to the examination, he may perform worse than his potential.

- Be creative when assessing a child with a brain injury. Standardized procedures often do not work well for children with impaired attention, arousal, motor abilities, or executive functioning. For example, most formal measures of visual construction use a score that is based on both speed and accuracy. You may need to assess visual construction ability only on accuracy when working with a child who presents with resolving motor paresis.

Gathering Data for Your Assessment

Given the child's age and developmental level, the reason for referral, and the type and severity of brain injury, you will need to plan an assessment using appropriate instruments and methods. Since performance on formal tests may overestimate or underestimate a child's ability to function "normally" within his regular environment, your conclusions should not be based on test findings alone. They should integrate a variety of information, including performance during formal testing, medical and academic history, behavior, and premorbid functioning. This information can be derived from sources, such as quantitative and qualitative data, clinical interviews and informal assessments, self and care-giver reports and questionnaires, your personal observations, background information, and hard and soft neurologic signs.

Quantitative and Qualitative Data

Both quantitative and qualitative test data are important to your assessment. *Quantitative data* is information measured or identified numerically. This type of data can be statistically analyzed and displayed visually in graphs and charts. *Qualitative data* is subjective data that is not numerical in form, which makes it more difficult to interpret. You can collect qualitative data using observations, interviews, and document reviews. Most comprehensive examinations use a combination of quantitative and qualitative techniques and data, which can allow for a more complete assessment of a child's functioning.

	Includes:	Is useful because:
Quantitative Data	• neurodiagnostic studies (e.g., CT, MRI, EEG) • norm-referenced scores, standardized rating scales • neurologic hard signs (See page 125.) • biological markers, such as microcephaly and abnormal chromosomes (e.g., Trisomy 21)	• School-age children and adolescents are usually familiar with taking formal tests. • Tests are administered the same way to all children of the same age. • Tests can be repeated to assess for changes in functioning. • Data can be presented in a format that is understandable by many different professionals.
Qualitative Data	• interviews • questionnaires • clinician observations • parent and teacher observations • process analysis of test performance. Process analysis relates to how or why a child may perform well or poorly on a task (e.g., a child may score within the impaired range because of poor attention, poor intellect, lack of effort, etc.).	• Many behavioral or emotional aspects of a child's functioning cannot be quantified. • A child's attitude, demeanor, and level of maturity are not easily quantified.

Discrepancies in quantitative data are sometimes explained by qualitative observations. The following case involving Diana is a good example of how qualitative information ultimately allowed us to accurately interpret Diana's data and make clinical conclusions regarding her difficulties.

Case Example 2 *Diana*

Diana, a nine-year-old, demonstrated good recovery from a TBI sustained during a boating accident. After Diana's discharge from the hospital, her mother began to complain that Diana was never able to complete her homework or school exams in the allotted time. During our examination, Diana demonstrated superior intelligence and seemed to have intact speed of *mentation* (i.e., how quickly she solved problems). Diana's scores on formal quantitative measures of processing speed (i.e., timed tests), however, were significantly lower than would have been suggested by her general presentation on other tasks. It was clear that Diana approached tests of processing speed differently than other tests.

Diana was extremely concerned with her accuracy when doing pencil-and-paper tasks of processing speed. She checked her work multiple times to make sure she did not make any errors, and therefore, was not able to complete as many items as expected. She did not have a problem with processing speed even though her formal scores were low. Instead, Diana scored low due to her insistence on checking her work for errors and not working as fast as she could (a speed-accuracy trade-off).

Clinical Interviews

Most information necessary to make a diagnosis is available through interviews. The information you gather can then guide the assessment, which may or may not confirm initial impressions.

The clinical interview is an important part of assessment. When assessing neurocognitive functioning, you can obtain a lot of useful information by asking questions similar to those presented below. Such questions can help you determine whether there may be specific deficits involving the child's behavior, motor skills, speech-language skills, executive functioning skills, etc.

Motor Skills
Can the child:
- button a shirt? sweater?
- zip his pants? jacket? (Pants are easier to zip than jackets because pants are fastened at the bottom of the zipper.)
- eat with a fork? spoon?
- use a knife?
- run? jump?
- walk up and down stairs? (Does the child use alternating feet on every other step, or does he use the more immature pattern, progressing one step at a time?)
- brush his teeth? his hair?
- tie his shoelaces?

Sensory Functioning
- Does the child wear glasses?
- Does he have difficulty hearing? (If *yes*, does the child come running when he hears his favorite TV show? If he does, the child may have an attentional or behavior problem rather than a hearing deficit.)

Executive Functioning
- Can the child pay attention to a variety of tasks (both favorite activities and difficult tasks)?
- Can he regulate his emotions and behaviors?
- How well does he adapt to changes in routine?

Speech-Language Skills
- Can the child maintain a conversation?
- Can he talk about both familiar and novel topics?
- Can he follow complex instructions?
- Is the child's speech intelligible?
  - Do persons familiar to the child understand his speech?
  - Do persons who are not familiar with the child understand him?

- Is his speech rate normal?
- Is his voice quality normal?
- What is his mean length of utterance?

Informal Interview Assessments

You can use informal interview questions, such as the following, to form an opinion about a child's mental status.

- What have you done today?
- Who are these people in your room?
- What did you eat for breakfast/lunch/dinner?
- What did you do last night/weekend?
- What was on TV last night?
- Why are you here today?
- What things do you find difficult since your accident?
- What do you do when you are hungry?
- What would you like to be doing one year from now?
- What do you need to do to achieve your goals?
- How did you get to this appointment? (for older adolescents)
- How did you remember to come to this appointment? (for older adolescents)

Often, a child will respond as if he remembers something, but he will actually be providing inaccurate information. Interview the parents or caregivers to confirm the accuracy of his information. When possible, and only once you have obtained the parents' permission, talk to other family members and teachers about the child. They may also share any additional problems or concerns they have noticed. Remember to ask open-ended questions to yield more information.

It is also important to ask the parents what they think their child's primary difficulty is. Once you have identified their main concern, assess for deficits relating to that concern as well as other areas that may cause similar problems.

Dr. John Walker, Dr. Lebby's mentor, used to say, "The parents are always right, although their reasons may be wrong. Finding out what is really going on is the first step in treating the child." Dr. Walker meant that it is important to listen to the parents because the information they give you is essential to your clinical assessment. He also realized that many times the explanation the parents give is incorrect. Even though the actual cause of the problem may be different from the parents' explanation, this does not decrease the importance of the information that they tell you in the interview.

Case Example 3 *Lateasia*

When Lateasia was 16, she was assaulted and severely beaten while walking home from school. She sustained an injury to the left hemisphere that affected her ability to process language. Lateasia's mother said, "Since Lateasia had the accident, she can't remember things." Her mother interpreted Lateasia's difficulties as a problem with memory functioning. After assessment, however, it became clear that Lateasia had no difficulty with memory functioning. Instead, she had enormous difficulty efficiently processing verbal and language-based information. Her difficulty with memory was only apparent when verbal information was provided too rapidly for her to process and understand. When verbal information was presented slowly in small amounts, Lateasia had no difficulty remembering it.

Problems with Interview Data Collection

Problems with data collection from an interview can arise from the following:

- Inadequate preparation of interview questions
  - Use a systematic framework to help you remember to ask important questions.
  - Pre-select questions based on history, diagnostic question, etc.

- Failure to appreciate the significance of a statement. For example, a parent may briefly mention that the child has difficulties making friends at school. Further questioning can reveal that the child has been bullied and his academic problems started around that time. This information helps explain why the child has difficulty functioning in school.
  - Probe to clarify information when necessary.

- Failure to notice inconsistencies in statements
  - Restate the information to the parent to make sure it is accurate.

- Missing the red flags that point to a specific deficit or problem
  - Pay close attention to the parents' concerns and ask questions as needed. Parents will often offer more information about the child's problem if you ask them to expand on their concerns.

Self-Reports and Questionnaires

Self-report measures and/or parent questionnaires are frequently used to determine the child's behavioral, emotional, and pragmatic functioning in a variety of environments (e.g., school, home, community). These tools can be extremely useful in an evaluation; however, non-critical acceptance of this data can lead to interpretive errors.

Errors from interview/questionnaire data are often related to:
- limited awareness on the part of the respondent (parent/caregiver/teacher)
- limited insight on the part of the patient
- emotional problems that interfere with communication of information
- poor ability of the patient to express or describe symptoms
- symptom exaggeration, minimization of problems, or malingering (i.e., deliberately faking a disorder)

Children with TBI often behave differently depending on the environment. For example, they generally perform better within a highly-structured environment (e.g., school). If the home environment is less structured, the child may exhibit more emotional and behavioral difficulties. Thus, when we send out questionnaires to a child's parents and teachers, the questionnaires sometimes contain different answers, giving different pictures of the child's functioning. Either the child acts differently at home versus school or the people interpret the child's functioning in different ways.

Behavioral Observations

Asking the child a few questions can give you a good initial understanding of his level of functioning. Additionally, much information can be obtained by observing a child's behavior. (See Appendix 7A, page 133, for a checklist you may use to record nonverbal communication behaviors exhibited by the patient.) Pay attention to the following when observing the child.

- Is the child oriented to person, place, time, and situation, or is he confused?
- How does the child interact with you? with family members?
- Does the child walk evenly or have a gait problem (e.g., limp, toe drop on one foot)?
- Are there physical limitations that may point to specific brain injuries?
- Does the child initiate conversation or wait until you ask him something?
- Does the child make eye contact and use facial expressions?
- Does the child appear anxious, nervous, depressed, or apathetic?
- How does the child attend to what is going on around him?
- Does the child have any insight into his difficulties?
- How does the child interact socially? Is it typical for his age?

Relevant History

The assessment should include information relating to the child's background. Using information about the child's school or medical history can often help explain a child's scores or performance. For example, a child who has difficulty reading may not have dyslexia, but instead, may have had very limited schooling. Knowing the child's background allows you to draw accurate conclusions and make appropriate recommendations.

- Review current and premorbid medical and psychological history.
- Review social, educational, and vocational history.
- Review relevant signs and symptoms relating to the complaint.
- Understand the nature of symptom onset and the progression of symptoms.
- Ask about the degree and nature of functional impairment.

Hard and Soft Neurologic Signs

Hard neurologic signs are easier to interpret than soft signs because hard signs give clear evidence of neurologic dysfunction (i.e., *pathognomonic* of disruption to central nervous system functioning). Soft signs are harder to interpret because they are correlated with, but do not confirm, neurological dysfunction.

Soft signs are not unusual for any child under eight years of age because soft signs are generally related to the functioning of an immature central nervous system. More soft signs, however, are seen in children with developmental disabilities or in those with a brain injury, than in children who are developing normally. It is also important to note that not all children with neurologic disorders will exhibit soft signs, and not all children exhibiting soft signs will have neurologic disorders.

Both hard and soft neurologic signs must be evaluated within the context and framework of your overall assessment. Hard and soft neurologic signs are difficult to interpret without additional information from your comprehensive evaluation. Diagnoses should not be based solely on the presence or absence of one or more neurologic signs.

Hard Signs

Hard signs include, but are not restricted to:
- abnormal infantile reflexes in non-infants (i.e., Babinski reflex, rooting, sucking, grasping)
- disrupted motor function in one or more areas (i.e., unilateral paralysis or weakness on one side of the body)
- disrupted sensory function in one or more areas (i.e., loss of vision in a visual field)
- dysarthria (slurred speech) that is not due to medications or physical injury
- apraxia of speech or limbs (inability to sequence motor movements)
- aphasia (loss of previously-acquired language skills)

Soft Signs (usually more diagnostic after age eight)

Soft signs include, but are not restricted to:
- hyperkinetic motor overflow (i.e., constant movement of extremities)
- impulsivity (e.g., the child responds prior to thinking or being given all of the stimuli)

- distractibility both internally (mind wanders/daydreaming) and externally (to environmental sounds and sights)
- inattention and difficulty focusing on one's work
- concrete thinking that is stimulus-bound (based on stimulus features), such as describing a bus as *something that is yellow and has wheels* instead of *a type of vehicle or means of transportation*
- simultaneous movements of opposite limbs or digits that are unintended based on the task
- uncoordinated movements
- immature grasp of writing instrument and difficulty drawing
- late milestone development
- slowed motor movements
- slowed processing speed (i.e., takes longer than usual to solve mental problems)

General Assessment Concerns

Due to the complexities of assessing children with TBI, you may find that problems arise that can result in error. It is important to know that:

- Errors can occur at all levels of assessment.
- Errors may be the result of carelessness, expediency, incompetence, or other factors.
- Errors may be serious or superficial.

You will be more likely to recognize errors if you review all of the quantitative data and compare it to your clinical judgment and qualitative information.

Errors in Testing

Evaluations are completed for many reasons, including the following.

1. determining eligibility for services and highlighting strengths and weaknesses
2. making treatment recommendations
3. evaluating the appropriateness of a specific diagnosis
4. stimulating discussion of potential problems that may arise later in development

Even under the best of circumstances, and even for experienced clinicians, the evaluation process can be challenging. You may encounter problems collecting and integrating adequate data, dealing with insufficient data, or interpreting data. Often, there is no perfect resolution, however, being aware of the problems and identifying them early may help you avoid making faulty assumptions due to errors.

Problems in Data Collection

- inadequate history or background
- inadequate behavioral observation during the assessment
- inadequate information derived from the assessment
- inadequate or inappropriate procedures used in testing (poor test selection)
- over-reliance on self-report or collateral reports (parent reports)
- over-reliance on formal test procedures
- errors in test administration and scoring
- failure to consider situational variables, such as time of day and distractions that may affect attention, motivation, and behavior
- failure to take into account the sample population from which a test was normed
- overemphasis on extreme scores that do not represent general functioning
- interpretation of scores within the normal range as being evidence of no brain impairment; a child's functioning may have dropped from superior to average due to the TBI
- failure to consider normal differences in performance
- failure to appreciate that everyone has strengths and weaknesses
- failure to compare the relevance of a test to everyday life
- report of global scores derived from many scores with a lot of scatter (inconsistencies in scores across subtests) without describing the intersubtest variability

Problems with Data Integration

Problems that can arise from data integration include, but are not restricted to, the following.

- lack of internal consistency (conflicting results)
- lack of external consistency (test scores conflict with the history)
- failure to take into account hierarchical nature of brain functioning
- failure to consider base rates for some syndromes, signs, symptoms (how often average people score the same as the tested child)
- failure to consider co-morbidity factors, pre-existing conditions, or other explanations
- overemphasis on establishing a formal diagnosis
- failure to take into account premorbid conditions such as subnormal intelligence, learning disabilities, prior head injuries, or medical problems that may be interfering with mental functioning

> The integration of test data with the interpretation of functioning is more important than the specific data generated by the testing. In other words, it is more important to know why a child did poorly on a test than the fact that he did poorly.

Problems Caused by Insufficient Data

A child may be referred to you by a parent who states that her child has "an attention problem." Your initial diagnostic impressions may lead you to believe that the child may have ADHD, which is common after a brain injury. By collecting more data from the parent, school, medical records, etc., it may become clear that the child really has a language-based disorder. Gathering more information helps you clarify the concern and allows you to plan your assessment accordingly. For infants, toddlers, and preschoolers, specific and thorough questioning regarding the child's development is very important, since school records are not usually available for this age group. Additional information will also be helpful when you have:

- *limited information available to support your conclusions and diagnosis*
  If test data indicates that a child with TBI has difficulty on verbal tasks, you may conclude that the TBI caused the difficulties. If you had more information indicating that the child always had language-based problems, your conclusions would be different.

- *a limited sample of performance to make conclusions*
  TBI most commonly produces inconsistencies in a child's ability to perform a variety of functional and cognitive tasks. When evaluating a child following a TBI, do not rely on only a few measures, as you may fail to fully appreciate the child's strengths and weaknesses. For example, poor performance on one test may not mean that the child has a deficit. The child may just have given a poor effort. Poor performance on several tests measuring the same skill gives more information regarding the child's difficulties. Conversely, good performance on a few isolated tests may not mean the child does not have a deficit, as shown in the following case example.

Case Example 4 *Vincenzo*

Vincenzo, a 14-year-old, suffered a severe brain injury when he was hit by a truck while riding his bicycle. Most areas of his brain were damaged, and he was in a coma, unable to interact with the environment for several months. Eventually, Vincenzo improved and was discharged from the hospital and allowed to return home.

During his one-year, follow-up neuropsychological evaluation, Vincenzo was still mostly unable to speak, walk, move his arms, or think independently. On most tests we administered to him, Vincenzo scored well within the impaired range, however, he did score in the high average range on a visual matrices test. The part of Vincenzo's brain that allowed him to solve visual matrix type problems was preserved.

128

Vincenzo, continued

Many tests of intelligence that use only one measure utilize a form of matrices to assess cognitive ability (especially those tests that are designed to be language and culture-free). If Vincenzo had been given a single test of intellect/reasoning that utilized a matrices-type measure, he would have appeared to have no cognitive problems and may have been described as functioning in the high average range of cognitive ability. This example highlights how giving only a few discrete measures of intellect to someone with a brain injury can be very misleading and should be avoided due to the variability in test performance in patients with TBI.

Problems with Data Interpretation

1. Do not assume that a brain injury in a particular area will cause problems associated only with the functioning of the area of the brain that has been damaged. Many children with TBI exhibit deficits that you may not expect, given the area damaged. Making assumptions based only on the brain damage results in predetermined expectations for the child's functioning and a tendency to test the child to confirm your initial expectations (confirmatory bias). You may inaccurately interpret the data by over-interpreting low scores or ignoring other scores when you have a bias. It is important, therefore, to remain open-minded to the specific deficits a child or adolescent exhibits regardless of his particular brain damage.

   We recently entered the room of an adolescent who had experienced a severe left hemisphere stroke, expecting him to be aphasic. He spontaneously initiated conversation with us, however, and exhibited only very subtle deficits with receptive or expressive language functioning. We have experienced many occasions in which a child's deficits do not match the specific pathology expected based on medical records or brain scans. The most important lessons to be learned from these experiences are:

   - No two children have the same brain anatomy.
   - Two children may have similar injuries but may present with different symptoms.
   - Two children may present with similar symptoms but their injuries may be in different areas of the brain.
   - Damage to the brain may not be expressed as functional impairment.
   - Significant brain damage may not show significant deficits in function.
   - Relatively small amounts of brain damage may show severe deficits in function.

2. Even though you may be able to generate an explanation for a child's specific cognitive deficits, performance, and/or behavior that fits all of the data, do not assume that your explanation is accurate. Seeing what you expect to see can cloud your judgment.

129

Dr. Lebby has often used the following axiom to teach his students about clinical interpretation and diagnoses and to help them understand their limitations.

■ *Explanation does not confirm etiology.* ■

This axiom suggests that just because you have a good explanation for something does not mean that you are correct about what is actually going on (the etiology). There are many plausible explanations for any one symptom. For example, a diagnosis of ADHD may fully explain the symptoms for a child who is fidgety, unable to concentrate, disruptive, and has limited ability to sit in a class for an entire hour. These same symptoms, however, would also be evident in a child with a language processing disorder who cannot understand what a teacher is saying. Therefore, the child could actually have a language processing disorder instead of ADHD.

3. Dr. Lebby also uses a rule he calls the *ipso-calypso rule* which is based on the logical reasoning of *ipso facto*. People assume that some things naturally lead from other things. In the case of a brain injury, it is easy to assume that any cognitive, behavioral, or emotional difficulty experienced by a child after a TBI is related to, or caused by the TBI. Therefore, it follows that if a child has difficulty with reading and he had a previous brain injury—ipso calypso—the brain injury caused his problem with reading. Sometimes, however, difficulties experienced after a brain injury have nothing to do with the actual injury. For example, the child's reading difficulties may have been related to an underlying developmental dyslexia syndrome and not the brain injury.

4. When interpreting data and the child's behavior, it is important to identify what is related to the brain injury and what is normal developmental behavior. For example, adolescents with brain injuries exhibit behaviors that are normal expressions of the need for independence and rebellion seen in other teenagers who have not experienced a brain injury. Therefore, behavioral difficulties in adolescents with TBI may simply be the adolescent "just being a teenager."

> Test data allows you to make assumptions about functioning. An assessment is just a snapshot of a child's functioning over a few hours in a controlled environment. Do not make absolute statements based on an assessment. Instead, use descriptive terms, such as "This suggests," "This is consistent with," etc.

5. Do not underestimate the potential of a child with TBI. Unfortunately, it is not uncommon to hear statements such as "He can't understand the information because he had a brain injury so there is no point in working with him." If you believe that every difficulty after a TBI is due to the injury, your expectations for the child's improvement will be lower than they would be if you consider that the behaviors or difficulties in question may be part of normal development. This view can result in excusing the difficulties and in believing that the child cannot improve.

6. When working with other professionals, be cautious about how therapies may impact testing results. For example, speech-language therapy incorporates many tasks that are similar to those used during a neuropsychological evaluation. If the patient was drilled on relationships between words in therapy, similar questions in a neuropsychological exam immediately following the therapy session may overestimate the child's level of functioning. Different results may be evident if the testing takes place several hours after the speech-language therapy session.

Test Selection

Many companies have developed specific tests for children of different age ranges, as well as for the assessment of different cognitive functions. At first, it may seem that test selection is the easiest part of the assessment; however, choosing the best tests for a specific need is actually more complicated than it first appears.

It is easier to determine which tests or combination of tests you should use once you understand the type of deficits expected, given the child's injury. Knowing the limitations and benefits for each test also makes it easier to choose which battery of tests to use. When determining which test(s) to use, consider the following rationale in your decision: *patient-independent issues* (relating to the assessment tools) and *patient-dependent issues* (relating to the patient).

Patient-Independent Rationale
Patient-independent decisions have nothing to do with the specific patient or client. They can include the following:
- examiner's familiarity and experience with the instruments
- availability of different instruments
- environmental constraints, such as time available to give the tests
- decisions about whether or not to administer the entire test, portions of several tests, or a combination of tests

Patient-Dependent Rationale
Patient-dependent decisions are based on the specific patient or client. They can include the following:
- information needed based on the referral question, clinical history, or described symptoms
- the age of the child
- the cultural background or primary language of the child
- the energy level of the child (how long can he tolerate assessment)
- medical or behavioral barriers that prohibit doing a longer examination
- motor or sensory limitations that make some tests inappropriate to give (e.g., tests requiring construction using blocks or drawings are inappropriate for a child who is paralyzed)

Determining the Length and Extent of an Examination

Over-testing can increase the chances that a child will fail a particular test, even when there is not a deficit with cognition. The chances for failure increase because there is some error built into tests, and performance varies due to behavior, fatigue, effort, etc. The longer an examination lasts, the more tired the child becomes and the less likely that you will accurately measure his best performance. Also, all children have relative strengths and weaknesses. Eventually, if given enough different tests, the child may fail one just because it measures something that he may not have learned.

Under-testing may result in a failure to adequately cover all of the relevant cognitive domains. Under-testing can lead to the clinician missing deficits or limitations and to a faulty assumption that everything is fine. Under-testing may also result in a clinician believing that if a child fails the few tests he is given, he is globally impaired. Further testing may demonstrate that the child has intact abilities in other areas of functioning.

Problems Encountered in Test Administration

Test administration is complex and involves many components. There are issues relating to test selection, data collection, scoring, and interpretation of the findings based on statistical norms. Because some responses may be unusual, clinical judgment is required when scoring a response and is always needed to interpret the data. There are many reasons why problems may arise as part of the testing process, including the following:

* lack of familiarity with standardized test administration leading to systematic error
* carelessness in administration (e.g., forgetting to administer easier items when the child does not achieve an appropriate basal score)
* conscious deviation from standard test instructions invalidates the norms (e.g., rewording questions or asking additional questions gives the child an advantage above and beyond those used to generate the norms)
* adherence to standard test instructions despite the need to adapt the test to allow the child to respond (e.g., failure to take into account the child's limitations or failure to make accommodations for disabilities)

Note: Professionals are encouraged to review the *Code of Fair Testing Practices in Education* to ensure that test administration follows the guidelines developed by the Joint Committee on Testing Practice. The Code provides guidance for both test developers and test users in four critical areas: (a) Developing and Selecting Appropriate Tests, (b) Administering and Scoring Tests, (c) Reporting and Interpreting Test Results, and (d) Informing Test Takers.

Code of Fair Testing Practices in Education. (2004). Washington, D.C.: Joint Committee on Testing Practices.

Child's Name _____

Date of Birth _____

Clinician _____

Today's Date _____

Pragmatic Behaviors Observed	Never	Sometimes	Almost Always
1. Hesitations/revisions	❏	❏	❏
2. Poor regulation of vocal volume	❏	❏	❏
3. Poor regulation of intonation	❏	❏	❏
4. Poor attending skills	❏	❏	❏
5. Delays before responding	❏	❏	❏
6. Inappropriate responses to questions	❏	❏	❏
7. Poor topic selection	❏	❏	❏
8. Poor topic maintenance	❏	❏	❏
9. Perseverates	❏	❏	❏
10. Problems with turn-taking	❏	❏	❏
11. Needs repetition of information	❏	❏	❏
12. Is gullible or naive	❏	❏	❏
13. Ignores social cues	❏	❏	❏
14. Lacks use of social graces	❏	❏	❏
15. Appears rude or lacks tact	❏	❏	❏
16. Hyper- or hyposensitive to environment	❏	❏	❏
17. Too much/little distance between people	❏	❏	❏
18. Difficulty understanding body gestures	❏	❏	❏
19. Difficulty using appropriate body gestures	❏	❏	❏
20. Poor eye contact	❏	❏	❏
21. Difficulty reading facial expressions	❏	❏	❏
22. Difficulty using facial expressions	❏	❏	❏
23. Difficulty with abstractions/jokes	❏	❏	❏
24. Difficulty with synonyms/antonyms	❏	❏	❏
25. Difficulty asking appropriate questions	❏	❏	❏

Chapter 8

Neurocognitive Assessment of the Child with TBI

Clinical assessment of brain functioning may seem daunting, but if you follow a relatively structured approach to your assessment, you will be able to readily assess many important aspects of neurocognitive functioning.

An assessment of functioning should include:

- relevant medical history
- pre-injury background and level of functioning
- interview and behavioral observation (can be the most informative)
- administration of formal tests (sometimes the tests need to be adapted or used in a non-conventional way)
- conclusions (provide diagnoses as appropriate)
- recommendations for a remedial plan
- attempted prognosis

An evaluation should include assessment and observation of:

- motor functioning
- sensory functioning
- attentional functioning (e.g., concentration, vigilance, impulsivity, distractibility, hyperactivity)
- language
- visual-spatial functioning
- verbal and nonverbal reasoning
- memory functioning (verbal and nonverbal/visual)
- associative and integrative skills (e.g., visual-motor integration)
- executive function and higher-order cognitive skills (e.g., problem solving, planning, self-monitoring, self-correction, generalizing, multitasking, switching mental sets)
- adaptive functioning
- affect, behavior, and motivation

Remember, recovery and loss of function change with time. Keep in mind that the results of the evaluation will vary, depending on factors such as:

- the date of the injury relative to the date of the assessment
- medical treatments the child is receiving
- medications the child is taking
- eating and sleeping patterns
- the age of the patient
- the time of day

Clinical Interview

We recommend that you begin your assessment by reviewing the child's medical history and then conducting a clinical interview (see Chapter 7, pages 121-123). The clinical interview will not only give you more information about a child's level of functioning, it will also help you:

- answer any remaining questions you may have regarding the child's medical history
- gain information about the child's developmental and functioning levels
- identify other factors that may affect the evaluation (e.g., whether the child slept well, ate breakfast, recently experienced a stressful event)
- obtain useful information to assist in the formulation of diagnostic hypotheses
- determine assessment needs
- plan the best way to administer the formal and informal components of the child's examination

▌Observations During the Evaluation

Formal test data is insignificant unless it is incorporated with other information about the child. Therefore, during your assessment, you should also observe and evaluate the child's emotional status, behavior, executive functioning skills, and his ability to perform complex tasks.

Emotion

A child's emotional status may significantly affect his performance, and ultimately your clinical impressions. The child's affective status should be considered as it relates to his motivation, effort, willingness to comply with testing, and his ability to perform at his potential during testing.

Case Example 1 *Mindy*

Mindy, a 13-year-old, was sitting on the tailgate of a pickup truck when the driver suddenly accelerated. Mindy fell from the truck, sustaining a skull fracture and subdural hemorrhage. A year after her injury, Mindy's testing showed significant deficits in most areas of functioning, especially attention and memory. Although this profile of deficits was consistent with her injury, we noticed a "red flag" that suggested an emotional problem instead of a problem with brain damage. We believed that Mindy's deficits might be related to her mood because her attention and memory were declining over time instead of improving post-injury. After a formal evaluation of Mindy's emotional state, it became apparent that she was clinically depressed. She was treated with psychotherapy and medications and her scores improved significantly.

Behavior

A child's behavior may also significantly affect his performance and your clinical impressions. Problems will arise if you fail to incorporate behavioral information into your diagnostic impressions. If you do not recognize the clinical significance of the child's behavior, you may interpret test results inaccurately.

Your assessment should also take into account the normal variability in childhood behavior. Keep in mind that a particular behavior may be normal at certain ages, but abnormal at other ages or developmental levels. For example, when we gave a four-year-old child a toy, he jumped up and down and flapped his hands in a stereotypic manner frequently seen in autistic children. In this context, however, it was clearly not pathological; it was an appropriate response to this child's excitement at receiving the gift. We also treated a two-year-old who exhibited echolalia. Although in an older child echolalia is suggestive of pathology, such as a transcortical aphasia or an autistic spectrum condition, it was appropriate for this child. Children naturally echo what they hear as a normal part of language development between 24 and 30 months of age.

A child's behavior can be considered abnormal when one or more of the following conditions is met:

1. The behavior is more intense than expected for the child's developmental age.
2. The behavior occurs more often than expected for the child's developmental age.
3. The behavior appears at a developmental stage when it would not ordinarily be expected.

Pay attention to the following when observing the child.

* level of effort, motivation, and arousal
* ability to sustain attention for several minutes at a time
* ability to process information without asking for it to be repeated
* ability to ignore distractions (internal and external), monitor his work, and self-correct when necessary
* receptive language skills—Does the child mishear words, frequently ask for information to be repeated, misunderstand instructions, etc.?
* expressive language skills—Does the child efficiently express himself, formulate verbal responses, organize sentences, etc.?
* speech skills—Are there any changes since the injury (e.g., dysarthria, apraxia, voice)?
* approach to problem solving—Does the child give up easily, become frustrated, or view difficult tasks as a challenge?
* flexibility of thought—Is the child perseverative, impulsive in his responses, or unable to process abstract information?
* consistency of the child's performance given the type and severity of the TBI—Inconsistent performance may suggest exaggeration of symptoms, malingering, or minimization of effort.

Executive Functioning

Assessment of executive functioning skills should involve formal and informal measures of the child's ability to initiate, navigate, plan, organize, and function within a complex environment. Executive functioning skills are independent of IQ, which relies predominantly on old learning and academically-based skills and knowledge. If a child has trouble with executive skills, he may need to be referred to a neuropsychologist for diagnosis and for assistance in treatment planning.

Flexibility of Thought

To test flexibility of thought, give the child a task to carry out, such as going to the hospital gift shop to get a newspaper or finding his room without any help. Finding familiar places within a large building like a hospital can be difficult for patients with poor executive functioning, even if they have normal IQ scores.

> Testing the limits of a child's performance gives more information than using relatively easy tests. Sometimes cognitive deficits only show up when a child is required to do challenging and complex tasks. Measures with low ceilings (most children are expected to perform well) may not give information about subtle deficits involving complex processes.

Case Example 2 *Sandy*

Sandy, a 15-year-old, sustained both a left hemisphere and a bi-frontal brain injury when a large rock fell on her head while she was rock-climbing without a helmet. As a result, Sandy lost her ability to use language and also presented with deficits in executive functioning, reasoning, and problem solving. We asked Sandy to find her way to a specific classroom at her high school, a familiar environment for her. Sandy wandered around the school without using any strategy to determine the location of the room. She finally wandered to a location directly in front of the room, but she failed to look at the room number. Because she didn't realize that she had found the room, she walked off in the wrong direction.

Sandy was unable to ask for directions because of her expressive aphasia. She also did not think about writing a question on some paper and using it to ask a teacher or the security guard for directions. In the end, Sandy became disoriented and frustrated and eventually began to cry.

Sequencing Skills

Determine if the child is able to follow a complex sequence of tasks without additional cues or prompts. Children with executive functioning deficits will have difficulty following a series of complex instructions because they may perseverate, make faulty assumptions, not pay attention to details, fail to plan ahead, or not notice and correct their mistakes. The clinical case example regarding Bryce in Chapter 5, pages 92-93, illustrates how a child with normal intelligence can have marked deficits involving sequencing skills.

Complex Skills

Complex skills rely on basic foundation abilities. Thus, problems with complex skills may be related to impaired basic functions. For example, a child with deficits involving drawing may have impaired vision, poor motor control, poor attention, or difficulty understanding the instructions. When a child has problems performing a complex task, break down the task into smaller components to see which specific skill or skills are impaired and which are intact.

Formal Assessment

Norm-referenced and standardized tests of neurocognitive abilities are available to a qualified examiner and should be utilized when detailed assessment is warranted. A relatively short screening examination may be all that is required to obtain a cursory understanding of a child's cognitive strengths and weaknesses. A comprehensive examination may not be practical given the child's level of functioning, ability to tolerate a lengthy assessment, or time constraints due to medication or therapy schedules.

Screening Neurocognitive Functioning in Children and Adolescents with the LANSE-C *and* LANSE-A

Drs. Lebby and Asbell have relied on their years of cumulative experience assessing children with TBI to develop two screening examinations that may be used to assess basic neurocognitive functioning within a clinical practice: the *Lebby-Asbell Neurocognitive Screening Examination for Children (LANSE-C)*, ages 6.0 – 11.11 years, and the *Lebby-Asbell Neurocognitive Screening Examination for Adolescents (LANSE-A)*, ages 12.0 – 17.11 years. In this section, they have also provided some useful information related to the screening of children and adolescents who have TBI.

It is important to remember that the *LANSE-C* and *LANSE-A* are not highly standardized assessments. They are, however, valuable tools for describing basic neurocognitive functioning and the behaviors of children who have had traumatic brain injuries. Using these assessments in conjunction with other screening tools should allow you to gather all the data you need for treatment planning. You can print copies of the *LANSE-C* and the *LANSE-A* for your personal use from the CD-ROM included with this book. Instructions and a Stimulus Book for each assessment are also included on the CD-ROM.

Use the *LANSE-C* and *LANSE-A* to assess the following areas of functioning. These screening tools will help you decide if the child needs further evaluation in a particular area and/or if you need to refer him to an appropriate professional, such as a neuropsychologist, speech-language pathologist, or neurologist.

Note: The *LANSE-C* or *LANSE-A* is not a substitute for a detailed, comprehensive examination of functioning, if one is required.

- General Functioning
  - motor functioning
  - visual and oculomotor functioning
  - hearing/auditory function
  - affect/mood
  - behavior
  - qualitative assessment of speech and language

- Level of Consciousness

- Orientation

- Attention
  - passive
    - sustained
    - number sequencing – forward
  - active
    - number sequencing – backward
    - number-letter sequencing

- Language
  - sentence repetition
  - receptive language (understanding verbal commands)
  - expressive vocabulary (confrontation naming)

- Reasoning
  - verbal associations
  - judgment

- Memory
  - verbal/auditory
  - visual

- Object Use

- Visual-Spatial Ability

- Visual-Motor Integration

- Visual Neglect

General Functioning

Review the patient's chart to get an idea of the child's general functioning level before administering the *LANSE-C* or *LANSE-A*. This information can help you know what to expect when you meet the child for the first time.

When you meet the child, make notes on the assessment form regarding his general functioning. You should also record the child's level of consciousness (i.e., alert, lethargic, apathetic, aggressive, or fluctuating).

If a child is ambulatory, we find it helpful to have him walk from the waiting room to the exam room. By walking with the child (if possible, walk behind him), you have the opportunity to observe his behavior and motor functioning. Watch to see if he walks with a limp or uneven gait, or swings one arm more than the other. You can also assess the child's ability to pay attention to you when there are external distractions and to see how well he follows directions. Be cautious when walking with a child who is recovering from a TBI, because children with TBI may be unsteady and have poor balance while standing or walking. Stay close to the child so you may assist him, if necessary.

Level of Consciousness

In medical records, the acronym *LOC* can be used to denote *loss of consciousness* and *level of consciousness*. You may wish to avoid using the acronym to reduce confusion.

A person's level of consciousness (LOC) can vary from normal (i.e., fully alert, talking, and making sense) to being deeply unconscious and not responding in any way, even to pain. There are many stages in between normal and unconscious. A patient recovering from a TBI may experience varying or fluctuating levels of consciousness from moment to moment or day to day. Therefore, it is important to make note of the patient's level of consciousness at the time of the *LANSE* screening. You can record the child's LOC by circling the appropriate level on the scoring chart. Use the following information as a guide.

- Alert—fully awake and appropriately responsive to internal and external stimuli; may have significant cognitive deficits despite presenting as appropriately responsive upon initial greeting

- Lethargic—not fully awake; may drift out of awareness when not being stimulated; may appear sleepy or confused with generally poor arousal or energy

- Apathetic—lacks motivation or initiation for goal-directed behaviors or volitional activities; shows diminished concern for things that were previous interests; exhibits loss of enthusiasm and spontaneity; may present as awake, but sits idly until someone gives him a direction

- Aggressive—characterized by irritability and a tendency for disinhibited verbal and/or nonverbal impulsive behaviors that may range from mildly disruptive to violent; often a temporary stage during recovery following brain injury

- Fluctuating—exhibits variations in level of awareness, energy, or appropriate responses and behaviors

Orientation

Orientation relates to the child's awareness of person (who he is), place (where he is), and time (date and time of day). If a child appears to be fully oriented, record the abbreviation *Ox3* (oriented times three) on the assessment. This indicates the child is oriented to person, place, and time. If a child is not completely oriented as expected for his age, write a short description of his abilities and limitations. The more information you can provide about a child's level of orientation, the better. The following are some examples of descriptions for a child's level of orientation.

> "Kathy is oriented to name but is confused about place and time. She accurately gave her name but stated we were at school and that it was 8 o'clock in the evening when it was actually 11 o'clock in the morning."

"Dashawn is oriented to name and place but is confused about time. He did not know the day of the week, date, or time of day."

"Alex was not oriented and presented as confused. He was unable to tell me his name, age, where we were, or the time of day."

If a child cannot tell time, adjust your expectations for his ability to judge time of day. Younger children should be able to answer *Is it daytime or nighttime?* and *Is it morning, afternoon, or evening?* For older children and adolescents, first present the question *What time is it?* If the child cannot answer the question, provide choices to see if the child is generally aware of the time of day.

Case Example 3 *Jeff*

Jeff, a 12-year-old, sustained a severe TBI when he crashed into a barrier while riding his ATV. Dr. Lebby had the following conversation with Jeff when completing the orientation section of a mental status exam.

Dr. Lebby: "Without looking at a clock or watch, about what time is it?"
Jeff: "Oh, hmm. I don't know what time it is."

Dr. Lebby: "Is it morning, afternoon, or evening?"
Jeff: "I'm not sure, but I think I just ate breakfast."

Dr. Lebby: "Do you think it is daytime or nighttime?"
Jeff: "I think it is daytime because I see the sun."

This example indicates that Jeff was not aware of the time but could make very general assumptions based on obvious cues. When possible, it is helpful to probe further to find out what the child is thinking and what kind of clues he needs to help him make sense of his environment.

Stating that a child is *Ox3* indicates he has basic orientation, but it does not fully measure any subtle or complex deficits he may have with orientation. Therefore, in addition to measuring basic orientation, we also ask questions to measure more detailed information regarding insight, demographics, and temporal awareness. Examples of questions that may assist in evaluating the child's functioning are:

- How old are you?
- When is your birthday?
- Who is that? (Point to a family member.)
- Why are you here?
- What happened to you?
- Where do you go to school?
- What grade are you in at school?
- What grades did you make on your last report card?
- How many siblings do you have?

- What is your mother's name? father's name? brother's name? sister's name?
- What did you eat for breakfast? lunch? dinner?
- Which is the first meal of the day—breakfast, lunch, or dinner?
- What is difficult for you to do since your illness/accident?

Attention

Screening typically involves assessing passive attention, sustained attention, and active attention.

Passive Attention

Passive attention is the ability to maintain focus on something that does not require mental manipulation.

▶ Sustained Attention

Sustained attention is the ability to maintain focus on an activity for an extended period of time. Given a stimulating environment and no significant distractions, a six-year-old child should have no difficulty working on tasks that are appropriate to the child's age or cognitive level (e.g., playing, watching TV, eating dinner) for up to 30 minutes without a break.

Following a brain injury, a child may only be able to sustain his attention for a few seconds or minutes at a time before needing a break. It is important to record the amount of time that a child can sustain his attention to a therapy session or examination in order to better schedule treatment, assessment, or school activities.

▶ Number Sequencing—Forward

A simple task that measures passive attention is to have the child repeat strings of numbers in the same order they are presented; however, number repetition is typically not appropriate for children under five years of age.

Number Sequencing – Forward	
By _____ years of age	Children should be able to repeat at least _____.
5	three digits
6	four digits
9	five digits
15	six digits

Active Attention

Active attention, or working memory, requires mental manipulation of information. Two tasks that measure active attention are repetition of numbers in reverse order and sequencing numbers and letters.

As children mature, their ability to manipulate information mentally improves. Very young children (approximately six years and under) rely more on rote learning than mental manipulation. After six years of age, children begin to develop the ability to think about and manipulate numbers and/or letters that they have already learned. If a child has not mastered numbers to ten and letters from A to Z, these tasks are not appropriate measures of active attention.

▶ Number Sequencing—Backward

A simple task that measures active attention is repetition of strings of numbers in the reverse order as presented (backward). Children should be able to repeat at least two numbers in reverse order by the time they are six, three numbers by the time they are eight, and four numbers by the time they are 15 years old.

▶ Number-Letter Sequencing

Active attention can be measured by asking the child to mentally sequence a list of mixed-up numbers and letters, and repeat them back to you with the numbers first, in numerical order, and then the letters in alphabetical order. Children should be able to sequence a list of three numbers and letters by six to eight years of age, and adolescents should be able to consistently sequence a list of four numbers and letters by 15 years of age.

Language

Assessing language is an important component of a general cognitive assessment. Screen for the child's general level of mixed receptive/expressive language (e.g., the ability to repeat orally-presented sentences), receptive language (his comprehension of spoken or written commands), and expressive language (the ability to express himself verbally).

Sentence Repetition

A child's ability to repeat sentences presented orally relies on both receptive and expressive language and speech skills. A simple task such as sentence repetition can give you some important information about a child's ability to listen, receptively process linguistic information, and communicate the verbal material via speech skills. Present increasingly longer and more complex sentences to the child, in order to determine whether the child's ability falls within age-expectancies or suggests a deficit involving language or speech skills.

Sentence Repetition	
By _____ years of age	Children should be able to repeat at least _____.
2 ½	two words (e.g., red ball)
3	three words (e.g., Cats say meow.)
4	five words (e.g., I like to eat candy.)
5	six words (e.g., The man has a big truck.)
6	seven words (e.g., Paul wanted a bike for his birthday.)

Receptive Language

To assess a child's understanding of receptive language, give the child simple commands to follow.

- Touch your nose (ear, arm, etc.).
- Wave good-bye.
- Point to your mother.
- Open your mouth.
- Look at the floor (ceiling, window, etc.).
- Blink your eyes.
- Spread your fingers apart.
- Point to the door (ceiling, window, floor, etc.).

If objects are readily available and are not distracting to the child, you may also give commands that ask the child to manipulate objects.

- Pick up the pencil.
- Give me the keys.
- Open the book.
- Put the crayon under the paper.
- Toss the ball to Mom.
- Turn the cup upside-down.

Finally, combine commands to determine if the child is able to understand complex commands.

- Touch your nose, then point to the window.
- Point to the book, then give me the keys.
- Look at the clock, then put the keys on top of the book.
- Open your mouth after you blink your eyes.
- Touch your ear, point to the ceiling, then wave good-bye.
- After you pick up the keys, give them to me and then point to the door.

Expressive Language

You can assess expressive language informally throughout your interactions with the child. Make notes regarding the child's articulation, voice quality, fluency, and general ability to express himself (i.e., syntax/sentence structure, sematics/content and word choice, and pragmatic skills/social appropriateness).

- Is the child able to tell you his name and respond appropriately to the orientation questions?
- Is the child's speech intelligible? If not, what is the problem (e.g., dysarthria, apraxia, articulation, paraphasic errors)?
- What is the quality of the child's voice and resonance?
- Does the child vary intonation, prosody, and inflection appropriately?
- Are the child's pragmatic skills appropriate given his age and the situation?
- Is the child able to describe a complex picture?
- Is the child able to converse about familiar topics?
- Is the child able to converse about novel topics?

Expressive Vocabulary

Assess expressive vocabulary by having the child name objects or pictures. Evaluate the child for *dysnomia* (difficulty in retrieving names). If a child is unable to name an object or picture, ask other questions to evaluate whether he recognizes the object and knows what it is. For example, you can ask, "Where would you find one of these?" or "What is this used for?" This will help ensure that the child's problem is dysnomia and is not related to limited exposure to the object or to *agnosia* (inability to recognize the object due to a visual processing deficit).

Reasoning

After a TBI, a child can have difficulty with reasoning and abstract conceptualization of information. A brain injury may cause a child to think concretely or in a stimulus-bound manner. For example, instead of saying that a dollar is a form of money, a child may say it is green, made of paper, or has a picture on it. A brain injury can also affect a child's judgment and safety awareness.

A child's ability to tell how two things are alike or similar (make logical associations) and answer questions that require good judgment can be screened with simple tasks.

Verbal Associations

Determine a child's ability to make associations between objects by asking him to explain how two objects are alike. Note whether the child gives a complex answer that indicates use of abstract thought or if he gives a concrete answer (i.e., a literal association regarding a feature of the item).

Judgment

To assess a child's judgment, ask him questions to determine his awareness of the appropriate course of action to solve everyday situations appropriate to his age. For example, you might ask:

- What would you do if you were locked out of your house?
- What would you do if your ball rolled into the street?
- What would you do if no one came to pick you up after school?
- What would you do if you found someone's wallet?
- What would you do if your friend told you to take something that did not belong to you?

If the child gives brief answers that do not contain enough information for you to determine if he understands the complexity of the situation, you will need to probe for more information. For example, you ask the child what he would do if his ball rolled into the street. If he responds, "Go get it," you should ask a follow-up question to make sure he understands that it could be dangerous to go into the street. You might ask, "Is there anything you should do before you go into the street to get the ball?"

Remember that even though a child provides an appropriate answer to a question, it does not mean that he will actually act in that manner if faced with the situation. Children with frontal lobe problems are especially susceptible to impulsivity, apathy, and inappropriate actions in social situations, even if they can explain what they should do in a particular situation.

Memory

Memory impairment, which is usually present after a TBI, affects almost all aspects of a child's cognition and functioning. It is difficult for a child to learn skills presented in therapy if he cannot remember the information. The ability to remember what is going on from day to day, or even hour to hour, helps a child become oriented to his situation and limitations.

The pattern of performance on memory tasks (free recall, cued recall, and recognition) is the same in children who have a brain injury and in children who have not had a brain injury. All children will find free recall tasks more difficult than recognition tasks that utilize true/false or multiple-choice formats. The scores for children with brain injuries, however, are often lower on each type of memory task when compared to their non-injured peers.

Verbal/Auditory Memory

Screen *verbal memory* by presenting three or four words to the child. Have him repeat the words until he can say them correctly (repeating the words twice is usually sufficient). Then ask him to remember the words. After fifteen to twenty minutes, ask the child to repeat the words again.

Testing free-recall memory without cues, recall memory with cues, and recognition memory allows you to better evaluate a child's memory ability. To test free-recall memory, you can ask a child to recall words from a list. You can give the child cues or hints, such as *One of the words was an animal*, to test cued recall. Finally, you can measure recognition memory by having the child pick an item from a list that includes the target word and foils.

Visual Memory

Screen *visual memory* by showing the child three or four objects. Allow the child to watch as you hide the objects around the room. After fifteen to twenty minutes, ask the child to tell you the names of the objects and where they are hidden. If it is too difficult for the child to tell you where the objects are hidden, you may allow him to point to them or even retrieve them for you.

Object Use

A TBI can cause a child to have difficulty comprehending basic object use. You can measure functional object use in several different ways.

- Say, "Show me what you do with this." Then give the child an object and see if he can pretend to use it appropriately. Use a variety of familiar objects, such as a toothbrush, cup, hairbrush, pencil, cell phone, and book.

- Pretend to use an object and ask, "Is this what this is for?" Use the objects in both appropriate and inappropriate (silly) ways to see if the child laughs or indicates that you are not using the object correctly. For example, place a cup upside-down on your head as if it were a hat, use a toothbrush to pretend to comb your hair, or pretend to brush your teeth with a hairbrush.

- Show the child several real or pictured objects, such as a pencil, a comb, and a cup. Ask the child, "Which one do you use to comb your hair?" or "Which one do you use for writing?" Have him choose his answer by pointing to the object. Some children may only be able to determine the accurate choice when you provide two choices. Others who are higher-functioning may be able to choose from a field of three or more objects.

- If the child is higher-functioning, show him a picture of an object and ask him to explain how the object is used.

Visual-Spatial Ability

A child with visual-spatial impairment may have difficulty recognizing things using only his vision (*agnosia*), locating objects in space, and/or judging the distance between himself and objects. When visual stimuli are distorted or have missing or covered parts, processing difficulties may become even more apparent. The following types of visual-spatial tasks will help you evaluate a child's ability to visually process objects.

- matching
- visual closure
- visual rotation
- visual organization
- figure-ground distinction
- matrices

Visual-Motor Integration

A child with impaired visual-motor integration may have difficulty drawing or writing. Assess visual-motor integration by having the child draw designs appropriate to his age. As the child draws, assess visual-motor functioning and look for errors in distortion, rotation, overlaps or gaps, proportion, and size.

Visual Neglect

A child with visual neglect syndrome will have a tendency to "neglect" or fail to attend to information within the neglected field. For example, a child may neglect food on one side of his plate, or objects to one side of him. You can assess neglect by having the child draw an object that should be symmetrical. Traditionally, neglect has been assessed by having a patient draw an analog clock face with the hands set at ten minutes to two. This technique works well for older children and adolescents who can tell time using a clock face. Have younger children draw a flower with petals and leaves to evaluate whether they neglect one side of the flower.

Chapter 9

Recovery Issues

With improvements in technology, children with TBI are living longer than ever before, but the amount and rate of recovery is different for each child.

Children recovering from an acquired brain injury present unique challenges to rehabilitative specialists, clinicians, and therapists. Recovery from a TBI can be as variable as the types of deficits caused by the injury. It can range from good recovery to very little improvement of functioning. Some children recover well enough to go back to regular education programs without significant difficulty, but even if a child with TBI regains premorbid levels of general functioning, subtle deficits often last indefinitely. The difficulties may not be obvious, but they can have a detrimental effect on the child's ability to function in a variety of situations. Mild difficulties may persist in the areas of multitasking, attention, memory, and learning. Ongoing limitations involving learning and memory can reduce the child's ability to maintain age- and grade-appropriate progress in school. The child may also have slowed processing, which can affect his ability to socialize with peers.

Brain recovery takes much longer than the recovery of other medical conditions (e.g., a broken leg). Although the rate of recovery can fluctuate, it usually starts quickly with most recovery taking place in the first six months post injury. Functional gains are still likely after six months, but they occur at a slower rate and can continue for many years following the injury. Slow and steady movement toward goals becomes the norm.

If children have deficits that last more than six months, the recovery of those deficits is likely to be incomplete because the brain has a limited ability to compensate for damage. Brain recovery is limited because damaged areas of the brain cannot produce new cells to replace those that die. There is some recent evidence that certain areas of the brain (e.g., the hippocampus) can produce new cells later in development, but the number of new cells appears to be extremely small and of questionable functional use.

The study of *neurogenesis* (i.e., growth of new neurons), especially that involving stem cells as a means of treating TBI and neuronal disorders, such as degenerative conditions, is in the very early stages of scientific research. This research is limited to animals and mainly involves highly-controlled areas of damage in the tissue of the central nervous system. At this time, there is little applicability of this research to the treatment of TBI in humans.

Families often misunderstand the meaning of recovery when it is applied to pediatric brain injury. They mistakenly believe that because a child's brain is not fully developed, he has a better chance to overcome a brain injury than an adult who suffers a TBI. For example, we met with the mother of a 13-year-old girl who was still in a coma almost six weeks after being injured in a motor vehicle accident. The mother assumed that because her daughter was injured at a "young" age, her brain would adapt to the injury and she would fully recover. It is true that immature brains that are still developing have more potential for recovery due to *plasticity* (the ability of the brain to change and compensate). It is also true, however, that an early injury can disrupt ongoing development of brain structures responsible for basic functioning, or more often, higher-level cognitive skills.

Deficits involving basic cognitive skills (e.g., language and visual processing) tend to show up relatively early following a TBI. Deficits involving more complex skills (e.g., the use of foresight, hindsight, planning, and organization; comprehension and expression of abstract concepts) may only become apparent much later, when the child has reached an older age. A young child may appear to show full recovery from a brain injury because he has returned to age-appropriate functioning, but the full extent of his deficits often does not become apparent until he matures.

▌ Processes of Recovery

Understanding the processes involved with the recovery of brain functioning can

> Cell growth involving axons and dendrites takes place slowly (roughly 1/1,000 meter per day), which partly accounts for the slow rate of brain recovery after an injury.

help you formulate opinions regarding the degree and type of plasticity and recovery you can expect to see in your patients. At the microscopic level, multiple processes take place to allow for brain recovery. Microscopic processes include:

- Cells in the brain produce new dendrite branches to make new connections with other cells.
- Previous cell connections are strengthened or altered to change how information is processed.
- Axon terminals change the amount of neurotransmitters that are released, making connections more effective.
- Axons produce sprouts to re-establish synaptic connections.

Unfortunately, there is a limit to the amount of recovery that can come from microscopic changes to cell structures. The reason for this is twofold.

1. Recovery only involves the cells that were undamaged in the injury.

2. With few exceptions, only the cells within the area of injury can help with recovery. Cells from undamaged areas of the brain generally do not take over functions for other damaged areas.

Cortical Organization

The simple analogy of brain cells to trees in a forest can help explain the processes involved with brain recovery. Brain cells have branches (dendrites), trunks (axons), and roots (axon terminals), and line up side-by-side just like trees in a forest.

Cellular Damage

Most brain injuries involve diffuse injury to axons over multiple areas of the brain (*diffuse axonal injury*). If the diffuse injury is mild, only some of the brain cells in an area will be damaged. This is like thinning a forest—some trees are removed but not all. At first, you will see the gaps in the forest canopy left by the removed trees. Within 6 to 24 months the remaining trees will grow additional branches to fill in the gaps.

The recovery of the brain follows a similar course. When diffuse injury thins cells, initially there are gaps in brain functioning related to the specific processes served by those cells. Over the next 6 to 24 months, the remaining cells grow more dendrites to fill in the gaps. These new connections overcome the disruption of functions that resulted from the injury.

A severe injury to a particular area of brain is more like "clear-cutting" a part of the forest. Clear-cutting leaves a large gap where trees used to be. The tops of the trees around that gap will never grow large enough to fill it in, leaving permanent areas of the forest without trees. In the brain, clear-cutting will leave permanent gaps in functioning that may never show recovery.

As discussed in Chapter 3, it is not expected that a person will recover 100 percent from a moderate or severe brain injury because, when vast numbers of cells die, the brain cannot fully compensate for the loss. In very young children, before the brain becomes organized into different functional regions, recovery can involve cells in distant areas. Once a child is more than a few years old, such compensation is much less likely and the chances of compensation by other areas of the brain declines.

As noted in Appendix 1A, page 25, Brodmann identified discrete areas of the cortex based on the types, staining properties, and organization of the cells. These areas have since been roughly correlated with functional regions of the brain. If there is clear-cutting of one of Brodmann's areas, it is unlikely that adjoining areas will take over the functions of the lost area because their cells and organization are different. This is like expecting an orange grove to begin producing apples if an adjoining apple orchard is clear-cut.

> **Case Example 1** *Samuel and Ron*
>
> Dr. Lebby has followed two patients with severe injuries to their language cortices for many years. Samuel had a stroke as a baby which resulted in the loss of most of his left hemisphere. This was Samuel's dominant hemisphere for language, so it would be expected that he would not develop language functions.
>
> Samuel, who is now ten years old, not only developed language functioning but has learned how to read, write, do mathematics, and is progressing well in school. Even though he has no motor cortex on the left side of his brain, he can walk and run and is able to dress and feed himself. Samuel's language functions were taken over by tissue in the right hemisphere, as were some motor functions for the larger muscles in his left arm and leg. He still has difficulty with fine motor functioning with his right hand and requires a brace to stabilize his right ankle. Samuel's language skills are functional but mildly delayed for his age with primary difficulties involving word finding and verbal formulation. Samuel has also developed a wonderful personality and sense of humor.
>
> Ron's injury was almost identical to Samuel's, but his recovery was very different. Ron suffered his stroke when he was ten years old. At 14 years old, Ron had not regained the ability to use functional language and still used pictures to communicate. Ron can produce a few single words and can recognize his name but is unable to use any connected speech to communicate. Unlike Samuel's brain, Ron's brain had already differentiated and developed into specific functional areas. When Ron had a stroke, the other cells could not take over the functions that were provided by the lost tissue.

Cumulative Damage

If a forest is thinned more than once, the ability of the remaining trees to compensate decreases, and eventually, there will be permanent gaps in the forest. Likewise, multiple diffuse injuries can cause cumulative brain damage that is equal to or worse than one moderate or severe injury. After an initial brain injury, there may be enough remaining brain cells to allow for recovery and compensation. Each additional injury, however, will cause more brain cells to die, which will ultimately result in gaps and permanent deficits in cognitive functioning.

With reduced cognitive functioning, the risks of additional injuries increase due to poor judgment, balance, or safety awareness. The net effect is that each new injury to the brain becomes more significant than the last, as a result of declining neurocognitive functioning and increased risk of further injury.

Predictors of Recovery

Although every brain injury is different, there are many similarities involving impairment and recovery in children with brain injuries. In general, outcome from a brain injury is related to three main variables.

1. physical aspects of the injury—This variable relates to the type of injury (open- versus closed-head injury), the severity of the injury (mild, moderate, severe, profound), and the extent of the injury (localized versus diffuse).

2. premorbid functioning—Children with healthy brains and typical intelligence before an injury often do better than children with premorbid developmental disabilities once the physical aspects of the injury are factored out.

3. support network and available resources—Children with supportive families and resources that allow for additional therapeutic activities or educational assistance after leaving the hospital generally recover better than children without such support or resources.

Accurately predicting recovery is most difficult shortly after the injury but becomes easier with time and as the child begins to show improvements in functioning. Unexpected outcomes do occur; therefore, you should be cautious when giving opinions about a child's expected recovery. We are cautiously optimistic when responding to questions regarding prognosis—always hoping for the best but preparing the child's family for the worst. Case Example 2 discusses two cases which resulted in different outcomes than initially predicted by the rehabilitation team.

Case Example 2 *Cortes and Mateo*

Cortes, a 14-year-old, fell from a fence and appeared mostly uninjured. Mateo, a 14-year-old, was involved in a high-speed motor vehicle accident in which there were several fatalities and appeared to be severely brain injured. The outcome of each child was very different, and surprised the staff on the rehabilitation unit.

Cortes rapidly declined in neurological functioning, and due to medical complications including increased intracranial pressure and seizures, eventually passed away from his injuries. Mateo made remarkable gains during inpatient rehabilitation and eventually returned to a regular school program. Mateo was fortunate to have few medical complications, well-controlled intracranial pressure, and no post-traumatic seizures.

Patterns of Recovery

Although children experience different patterns of recovery, as a group, they appear very similar. Some similar patterns of recovery are:

- Children with more severe injuries are less likely to improve over the first two years following an injury than children with less severe injuries. Measuring a child's recovery past two years becomes difficult because it is often not possible to separate recovery from new learning and development of new skills.

- Children progress through similar stages of recovery; however, the progression can vary significantly from patient to patient. Some patients will pass through most stages, others may skip one or more stages, and others may progress to a certain stage and then plateau. Recovery may take days, weeks, months, and sometimes a year or more, with less recovery as time passes.

- Children may go through multiple periods of rapid gains followed by days or weeks of little recovery. The phrase "turned a corner" is often used to communicate that a patient is beginning to show consistent and measurable gains following a period of little improvement. In most cases, a child will turn many corners as he goes through several periods of rapid recovery followed by periodic plateaus.

- Rate of recovery varies due to reasons such as:
  - medical complications
  - pain (It has become standard practice to assess a child's level of pain, as part of an examination.)
  - fatigue
  - attention deficits
  - motor limitations
  - frontal lobe dysfunction

Stages of Recovery

The *Rancho Los Amigos Levels of Cognitive Functioning (RLA)* is a classification scale used by clinicians to assess and monitor recovery of neurocognitive functioning in rehabilitation patients with TBI. The model was developed at the Rancho Los Amigos National Rehabilitation Center in California, and is widely utilized in rehabilitation centers and hospitals. A copy of the scale is included on the enclosed CD-ROM.

The *Rancho Los Amigos Scale* consists of eight levels used to describe the stages of neurocognitive recovery typically observed in patients after a brain injury. For most patients, the stages of recovery from a TBI closely match the levels on the *Rancho Los Amigos Scale*. The stages of recovery, with their corresponding RLA scale values, follow along with additional information that is helpful to those who work with patients with TBI.

RLA Stage I—The child does not respond to stimulation (auditory, visual, or tactile).

RLA Stage II—The child responds to stimulation, but only in a general manner (i.e., increased arousal, moaning, or increased tone to stimulation).

RLA Stage III—The child demonstrates some localized responses to stimulation, such as rubbing where it hurts or pulling at tubes. He often has inconsistent arousal and may be able to follow some simple commands inconsistently when he is alert.

▶ Author Recommendations for RLA Stages I, II, and III

- Treat the child with respect. Remember the child is a person first and a person with a brain injury second.

- Cover exposed body parts that would make the child uncomfortable if he was aware of his situation.

- Talk to the child in a normal voice as if he understands you. Even though he may appear to be asleep, he may be able to hear what is going on in the room.

- Restrict the number of visitors and keep noise levels low to prevent agitation. The child will often respond to different levels of stimulation within the room.

- Be alert for behaviors that may indicate the child is in pain or is uncomfortable (e.g., increased restlessness, agitation, moaning, etc.). If you identify such behaviors, consult members of the treatment team who may be able to help the child.

- Keep therapy sessions relatively short to prevent increased agitation. Even a few minutes of stimulation can be overwhelming to a child during RLA stages I through III.

- Recommend that family members get some rest and take care of their own needs. This is often a difficult time for family because the prognosis for outcome may not be very clear. As the child wakes up from a coma and is more able to tolerate therapy, the family's involvement will increase.

- As the child becomes more aware of his environment, speak to him in short sentences. Simple directions, such as *Squeeze my hand* are appropriate, while two-part commands usually overwhelm the child.

- Wait at least 30 seconds after giving a direction before assuming that the child did not understand your instruction. The time it takes the child to give a response or follow a command may seem long, but that is expected.

- Make sure the child receives periods of undisturbed sleep during the day and longer periods during the night. Rest is important for patients at these stages of recovery.

- Monitor the child's sleep patterns and facilitate regular sleep-wake cycles as he progresses.

RLA Stage IV—The child may have increased arousal but with agitation and restlessness, usually due to discomfort or confusion.

RLA Stage V—The child is often calm without excessive restlessness or agitation. Confusion and post-traumatic amnesia persist, disrupting awareness and orientation. The child may be inconsistent with object use or when following directions. There are no goal-directed behaviors, and the child's functioning is dependent on external prompts. The child may have little, if any, awareness of his deficits and no ability to act safely due to impaired awareness and judgment.

▶ **Author Recommendations for RLA Stages IV and V**

- Minimize agitation and restlessness by keeping stimulation to a minimum when you are not working with the child.

- Communicate with the child using short, positive statements. Use simple words that are directly to the point. For example, ask, "Are you in pain?" instead of, "How are you feeling?"

- Assume that the child does not remember you. Introduce yourself each time you encounter the child for assessments of therapy. Explain who you are, why you are there, and what you would like him to do. Help the child understand his situation by saying things like *You are in a hospital*, *I am going to show you some picture*s, and *Tell me what you see here.*

- As the child's cognition and memory improve, provide prompts and cues to help him find the right answer. Providing cues will allow the child to be successful and will help reduce his frustration.

- Talk to and treat the child at a level that is age-appropriate. For example, avoid treating an adolescent with a brain injury in the same manner you would treat a five-year-old. Although the adolescent's cognitive deficits are apparent, he will have more pre-injury experience and will retain much of his old learning.

RLA Stage VI—The child is able to use objects appropriately and has goal-directed behaviors. Confusion persists as does post-traumatic amnesia, but these conditions are not as severe as they were for level IV. The child is able to follow a schedule but requires external cues and prompts. Awareness of primary deficits emerges, but awareness of more subtle deficits is often limited. Safety awareness and judgment remain deficient.

RLA Stage VII—The child may have regained most of his cognitive functions with the exception of executive functioning. Memory for day-to-day activities is relatively functional within a structured environment, but may be deficient for less-structured materials, such as a list of facts. The child is able to function independently within a highly-structured environment where therapists and staff organize the day. Foresight and hindsight remain impaired but awareness of deficits may be mostly intact. Safety awareness and judgment is adequate within a structured environment but may be deficient in a more complex environment.

▶ Author Recommendations for RLA Stages VI and VII

- Demonstrate the child's ongoing deficits to family members to help them understand the need for increased supervision and attention. Many patients at levels VI and VII appear to function well during bedside conversations. Thus, family members often overestimate their cognitive abilities.

- Use simple, positive phrases and statements. This will be beneficial to the child as he may continue to have ongoing confusion.

- Avoid using abstract concepts, negative statements, or complex linguistic forms (i.e., sarcasm, innuendo, analogies) as the child's thought processes are often concrete and stimulus-bound.

- Give the child a break or alternate the type of therapy he receives every 30 minutes. For example, follow speech therapy with occupational therapy and/or physical therapy. Then, the child may be able to tolerate another session of speech therapy or he may need to take a break and rest.

- Provide semantic and physical cues when a child has difficulty responding to a question. Word-finding difficulties, which can result in frustration and reduced cooperation, are often evident at these stages of recovery.

- Have the child keep a memory log. Memory logs are beneficial during these stages because they help the child remain oriented to day and time, and they allow the child to review his routines and make sense of his daily activities. Continue to use memory logs as long as the child presents with memory deficits.

- Remind the child about his limitations to help him develop better insight. A child can work toward becoming more independent if he has a better understanding of his strengths and weaknesses.

- Encourage the child to continue doing things for himself as he becomes more automatic in his daily routine.

- Evaluate and provide therapy in less-structured environments where executive functioning deficits may be more evident.

- Talk about what the child has done during the day to help him integrate past and present.

- Discuss goals and help the child understand how his current functioning will impact his future functioning. Discussing goals on a regular basis will facilitate the child's progress.

RLA Stage VIII—The child is able to integrate past, present, and future. He has a good awareness of his limitations and deficits, and how they will impact his life. Judgment is mostly intact, allowing for independent functioning. Subtle deficits, however, involving executive functioning, memory, social skills, and more complex academic abilities involving abstract conceptualization of information may persist. New learning may be disrupted, although basic cognition may have recovered to age-appropriate levels.

▶ Author Recommendations for RLA Stage VIII

At stage VIII, return to school and an age-appropriate social environment become important. A child may require accommodations or resource services at school now that he has new physical and/or cognitive limitations. Language and executive functioning deficits may continue for many years, and may interfere with age-appropriate social activities. Once the child realizes that some of his deficits may be long-term, he may experience increased frustration and depression.

The child may need help "fitting in" with peer groups. His social inadequacies may make interactions with his friends awkward. Many patients eventually stop socializing with their friends because it becomes too difficult for them to keep up with conversations. They also may not get jokes or recognize subtleties in their friends' facial expressions or tone of voice.

- Teach the child ways to help him overcome higher-order language and communication problems. Work on social and communicative reciprocity, turn-taking, and following a theme or idea.

- Help the child understand his ongoing weaknesses and teach him how to compensate or accommodate. For example, if he has problems with executive functioning, teach him how to take more efficient classroom notes, use a tape recorder, or organize his homework.

- Work on skills, such as using mnemonics or acronyms, to help the child remember information.

- Teach the child to write notes about things he needs to remember so he does not forget important information or activities.

- Teach the child patience so that he does not expect instant recovery or become overly frustrated with ongoing deficits. Help him understand that he will likely have ongoing recovery for many months or years.

- Build the child's self-esteem and confidence by reminding him of his strengths. Show him how to use his strengths to overcome his weaknesses.

- Reward the child's efforts as well as his successes.

Hospital Course During Recovery

Hospitalization after a TBI and during recovery involves different departments and levels of care. Multiple specialists, as well as family members, may be involved in the patient's care and recovery process. Appendix 9A, pages 170-171, provides a list of interdisciplinary team members who are typically consulted during the child's hospitalization and rehabilitative course.

The typical course of hospitalization involves five stages—emergency department, intensive care unit, acute medical rehabilitation unit, community reintegration, and discharge home. These stages correlate with physical changes in the brain resulting from the trauma and processes of recovery. They also encompass the many emotional periods and events experienced by the patient and his family.

It is helpful to compare the parents' emotional state throughout the child's recovery to the process of grieving. They grieve not for the loss of their child but for the loss of what their child could have become or achieved. Although a family's early

> Improvement continues for many years following TBI. A child may not achieve his potential if therapy is stopped too soon.

response to injury can prevent them from adjusting to their situation, acceptance of the permanence of limitations and the changes that must take place can ultimately lead to improved emotional stability.

Stages of Recovery

Stage 1—Emergency Department

At the time of the injury, many physical changes occur in the brain. Some are related to the actual trauma. Others are secondary processes caused by disrupted normal functioning of the neural systems. These can include bleeding (*hematoma*), loss of oxygen (*hypoxia*), cell death (*ischemia*), and/or swelling (*edema*). If brain swelling becomes too severe, the pressure can force brain tissue across membranes (*herniation*) which is life-threatening if untreated.

Damage to the brain can result in the release of neurotoxins and excessive amounts of neurotransmitters, such as *glutamate*, which can damage additional cells. Because the brain requires a delicate balance of chemicals, such as electrolytes, to function, disruption of this balance due to brain injury can become life-threatening.

During this period, the patient receives intensive medical intervention that often includes airway management. The treatment team becomes focused on the patient's medical needs required to sustain life and may be unable to communicate with family members. Family members frequently feel like they have been "left out of the loop," which can lead to anxiety, fear, confusion, and panic. Parents may feel a loss of control, often combined with guilt, and may experience increased distress and anxiety if the child's condition does not quickly improve.

Stage 2—Intensive Care Unit

This stage varies depending on the severity of the injury, medical complications, and the length of coma.

Once the child is admitted to the intensive care unit (ICU), any ongoing damage to the brain from problems, such as swelling, are brought under control. This may take several weeks, so it is important that the child be allowed to rest and recover quietly during this time. Reduced stimulation allows for improved recovery as most kinds of stimulation at this stage of recovery have the potential of raising the child's blood pressure and/or intracranial pressure.

From a family perspective, this can be the most difficult and frightening time of recovery. Things happen quickly in the ICU, and parents have little control over their child's care. While the child remains in the ICU, the parents may have limited access to him, and when they do spend time with their child, he may be unconscious and connected to machines.

Families often have questions that cannot be easily answered by medical staff due to the fragile nature of the child's condition. The staff must guard the child's prognosis and respond to questions cautiously due to the unpredictability of the child's outcome.

Parents tend to react emotionally because there is little to do other than sit and think about the situation. They generally spend many hours in waiting areas with one salient concern, "Will my child recover?" Feelings of helplessness, confusion, frustration, and fatigue develop from not knowing the prognosis. The parents' emotions may also be compounded by stress and lack of sleep.

Stage 3—Acute Medical Rehabilitation Unit

Once a child is awake and medically stable, he may be moved to a rehabilitation unit. Demands on the child will be slowly increased so that he can begin to participate in *activities of daily living*

(ADLs). In the early stages of rehabilitation, it is more important that the child is engaged in activities (i.e., doing something) rather than what those activities are.

The move to a rehabilitation unit offers relief for parents because their child has made it through the life-threatening stages of his condition. The move, however, is also a time of realization for parents. Previously, they were isolated from the day-to-day activities surrounding their child. Once a child begins rehabilitation, parents are expected to become active participants in his care.

Parents should be encouraged as early as medically possible to establish standard daily routines. They should make sure their child has regular wakeful and sleeping hours and keep him busy throughout the day so he is tired at night. This may sound simple, but the majority of children with TBI will experience physical, emotional, and behavioral changes that hinder adjustment to recovery and rehabilitation. Pain, emotional lability, agitation, irritability, confusion, frustration, memory deficits, reduced level of tolerance, and/or lack of cooperation can all get in the way of a child's progress. This is especially true for children who are over-indulged by their parents.

Rehabilitation is an emotional time for parents. Their defenses break down, and they begin to express their previously inhibited thoughts and feelings of anger, frustration, and guilt. Up until this point, parents' expectations for recovery were often exaggerated by optimism, denial, and wishful thinking. Now their hopes for a full recovery are replaced with the realization that their child will have long-term deficits. The patient's and family's focus shifts from "getting back to normal" to short-term therapy goals, such as the following:

- Speech and language goals may include gaining the ability to vocalize, then to verbalize, and ultimately to communicate.

- Physical therapy goals may include the ability to take a step or even sit unassisted.

- Cognitive goals may include improved awareness of the environment or the child's deficits.

- Basic goals for being as independent as possible in activities of daily living replace premorbid expectations.

The type of injury (i.e., severity and area damaged) and the child's personality characteristics play roles in the reaction the child has during recovery and rehabilitation. It is not possible to predict how a child will react to the rehabilitation process. Children who were previously very competitive and very active may become passive and apathetic, while others who were more reticent have surprised us by exceeding every goal set for them. Parents, caregivers, and therapists should work on expanding the child's retained functions, in addition to optimizing participation, by taking advantage of his strengths.

Case Example 3 *Celiena*

Celiena, a 15-year-old, contracted an infection of her brain and spinal cord. When Celiena came to the rehabilitation unit, she was not able to lift her head or move her limbs. Her cranial nerve damage resulted in facial paralysis and visual problems. When she sat up, she would become dizzy, throw up, or even pass out. At first, she didn't want to be in rehabilitation but soon began to work extremely hard during her therapy sessions. By the time she was ready to be discharged home from the rehabilitation unit, she was walking short distances without the assistance of braces or a walker.

The day before being discharged home, she wrote the following:
I've left the dream world behind. Everything happened so fast, it was basically like a dream. Seventy-two days in the hospital is enough for me. My health is good. I continue to experience improvement every day. I can expect the daily tasks like getting dressed, which so many of us take for granted, to become easier as time goes on. I still need a wheelchair for long distances. What I learned from my experience is you have to believe in yourself and never say, "I can't do something," because you can!

Stage 4—Community Reintegration

To facilitate successful reintegration into the community, inpatient rehabilitation programs should incorporate outings that expose the patient to less-structured environments. Therapists should integrate activities that are representative of the child's home life, such as making a purchase in the gift shop, ordering food in the cafeteria, shopping for music CDs, picking out clothing, or simply navigating around a large store. For children in wheelchairs, therapists should also include activities that involve navigating parking lots, curbs, and narrow store aisles.

Stage 5—Discharge Home

Discharge from an inpatient medical rehabilitation unit can be a mixed blessing for the patient and his family. Over the months of rehabilitation, the family has developed bonds with the medical and support staff, and they have come to rely on the structure and support the staff provides as part of the rehabilitation program. Although most families look forward to going home, leaving such a program also results in feelings of loss, anxiety, and even abandonment.

Throughout rehabilitation, children often make steady gains in functioning. This progress leads parents to hope that recovery will continue until their child has regained most, if not all, premorbid functioning. As the discharge home date approaches, reality begins to set in. Parents must reconcile the fact that the acute stage of rehabilitation is coming to an end, and their child will most likely have long-term deficits.

As their child prepares for discharge home, parents have many decisions to make. If their child has ongoing motor limitations, they will need to make decisions regarding adaptive devices, such as the color of a wheelchair or if their child needs bathing equipment and/or medical supplies. If their child has cognitive deficits, school re-entry becomes an imminent concern. The realization that special education resources are now required may be traumatizing for parents who had hoped for a more complete recovery.

Recovery tends to slow substantially after patients are discharged from rehabilitation. Gains become obvious on a weekly or monthly basis instead of day-to-day as was evident early in rehabilitation. Cognitive deficits, especially those relating to executive functioning, may become more evident when the formalized support and the structure from the rehabilitation team are removed. Patients, who have mastered the daily routine of their therapy program, may become overwhelmed when faced with the complexities of an environment outside the rehabilitation setting and may fail to complete even simple tasks.

Case Example 4 *Ashley*

Ashley, a six-year-old, sustained a brain injury when she was hit by a car as she ran across the road. In the rehabilitation unit, Ashley appeared to recover at a rapid rate and soon regained the ability to talk, understand conversations, and wheel herself around in her wheelchair. She clearly enjoyed the wheelchair races she had with the staff and the authors. The races became a part of Ashley's normal routine, and her wheelchair skills improved quickly. When Ashley went home, however, her affect, behavior, and emotional state changed dramatically. She wanted to play with her friends who were running around and soon became frustrated with her chair. When Dr. Lebby spoke to her mother, she reported that it seemed normal to Ashley to be in a wheelchair when she was at the hospital because there were other children in chairs and the staff frequently used chairs during therapy sessions. At home, Ashley was the only child in a chair. The realization that she could not play with her friends in the same way as she used to was emotionally traumatizing for her.

As in Ashley's case, transition home from the rehabilitation unit can be as difficult, if not more difficult, than life on the rehabilitation unit, especially for young children with permanent disabilities. Most children adapt well to their new deficits, especially for the first year or two when changes are still evident and recovery continues at a slow rate. A year or two after discharge, however, some patients experience a decline in their functionality. This decline is rarely related to brain deterioration. It is generally the result of emotional and psychosocial factors that come from the child's realization that his deficits are likely permanent and will have compounding social ramifications. Children with brain injuries frequently lose friends and have trouble making new friends. They are viewed as different or difficult to include in activities due to their physical and/or cognitive limitations. Given these issues, a child may experience depression and should be monitored by his parents and medical professionals.

▶ Cognitive Deficits Post-Discharge

The family's social background and available resources should be considered when making recommendations. Do not develop a treatment plan that is overwhelming or that cannot be achieved by the family, as they are less likely to follow it.

Frequently, a child is discharged from the hospital once he is walking and able to take care of basic activities of daily living. Although the child may look, act, and interact as if he is completely recovered, he may still have significant cognitive deficits. Recognizing these "hidden" deficits is crucial in advocating for the child. It is also important to identify the child's cognitive strengths and weaknesses in order to provide appropriate therapy and accommodation recommendations that will facilitate participation when he returns to school.

Case Example 5 *Vanessa*

Vanessa, a 16-year-old, was severely injured when she fell from a roof onto a concrete driveway. She sustained a severe closed-head injury with multiple intraparenchymal hemorrhages. Vanessa recovered relatively well while in the hospital but left the hospital with notable, ongoing cognitive deficits. She recovered her basic intellect and academic skills quickly, and by four months post-discharge, her scores had returned to a level just below the average range. By one year after discharge, her intellectual and academic scores had returned to the average range.

Vanessa's recovery of memory and executive functioning took much longer and did not recover to the same degree as her intellect and academic abilities. After a year post-discharge, Vanessa's memory and executive functioning scores still fell within the impaired range for her age, even though they were slightly higher than when she left the hospital. This pattern of recovery is quite common, with relatively rapid return of basic cognitive functions and slower return of more complex and integrated functions, such as executive abilities and memory.

Vanessa's memory difficulties make it difficult for her to learn new information in a classroom setting. Her memory deficits are especially evident when material is complex, when she must remember unstructured facts (e.g., a list of state capitals), and when she takes recall-type tests. Recognition tests using a multiple-choice format are easier for Vanessa, although she still has some difficulty with them.

Vanessa's executive functioning deficits make it difficult for her to process information quickly, multitask, switch mental sets, and maintain her attention for complex information. In the classroom, these limitations cause her difficulty in keeping up with lectures (slow processing speed), writing notes while listening to her teachers (multitasking), and switching from writing notes to listening or from one thought to another (switching mental sets). Vanessa would be able to function much better in the classroom if information was presented serially and she had time to complete each component before moving on to another.

Results of Vanessa's Neurocognitive Evaluation

Cognitive Function	At Discharge	4 Months Post-Discharge	12 Months Post-Discharge
Verbal Reasoning (VIQ)	60, 0.4% (deficient)	84, 14% (low average)	98, 45% (average)
Visual Reasoning (PIQ)	55, 0.1% (deficient)	75, 5% (borderline)	102, 53% (average)
General Intelligence (FSIQ)	54, 0.1% (deficient)	77, 6% (borderline)	100, 50% (average)
Memory Recall	1-4 (deficient)	1-4 (deficient)	1-5 (deficient)
Executive Functioning	1-2 (deficient)	1-3 (deficient)	1-4 (deficient)
Reading Composite	78 (deficient)	95 (average)	105 (average)
Mathematics Composite	75 (deficient)	98 (average)	100 (average)

In young children who are hospitalized for many months and continue to have deficits for many years, there may be a delay in emotional and behavioral maturation. Young children with TBI can be physically and cognitively dependent on parents/caregivers for several years. Being dependent on others can result in a child failing to develop age-appropriate independence, confidence, and self-esteem. The child may not have had the opportunity to succeed or experience the transition from dependency to independency because of his inability to function alone.

Even though the child may be at an age where independence and self-confidence normally develop, the deficits from the TBI may prevent this from happening. Behavioral and emotional immaturity are often evident after a brain injury because of damage to the brain (i.e., disrupting brain development) and as noted above, because the child's deficits make him more dependent on others.

Safety Concerns

Following his discharge from the hospital, a child with TBI may still have many subtle deficits in thinking ability. He often does not exercise concern for his safety or the safety of others. He may act and behave impulsively due to an inability to self-monitor and regulate his behavior. In addition, he frequently may show impaired or diminished judgment, which can result in him doing dangerous things or not recognizing when he is in a dangerous situation. All of these factors increase the risk of a second injury.

The child's lack of safety awareness imposes a duty upon those who care for the child to exercise a high degree of vigilance and caution and to provide more stringent structure and boundaries for safety. They must protect against additional injury by being aware of risk factors, such as the following.

- poor balance and coordination

- risky sports activities that can result in an injury (e.g., football, diving, boxing)

- risky recreational activities that can result in injury (e.g., skateboarding, skiing, snowboarding, motor-cross, dirt bike riding, ATVs, snowmobile riding)

- higher risk for bullying or victimization

- the use of recreational drugs and alcohol

In a person with a brain injury, the effects of drugs and alcohol increase because the parts of the brain that control reasoning, judgment, and motor coordination are already disrupted. The extra disruption from the drugs and alcohol can result in significantly increased levels of impairment.

▌ Medication Considerations

Medications may allow for improved functioning in a child recovering from a TBI. Medications are most commonly prescribed when the child has difficulties, such as the following.

- excessive fatigue
- reduced arousal
- poor attention
- behavioral impulsivity
- social disinhibition
- affective/emotional disruption (i.e., depression and anxiety)

When prescribing medication, the focus should be on treating the symptoms, not the disorder (TBI). When making a decision regarding whether medication management is appropriate for a child, ask the following questions. The answers will help determine if safety, learning, and/or emotions are areas of concern for the child.

- **Safety**—*Is the child at risk for hurting himself or others?* Medications can help a child control his behavior.

- **Learning**—*Does the child use the majority of his resources to compensate for attention difficulties or to stay awake, and have little energy left for actual learning?* Medications can assist in increasing a child's ability to focus his attention. They can also increase his arousal level to help compensate for lack of energy and fatigue.

- **Emotions**—*Is the child excessively depressed or apathetic, and, therefore at risk for failing at school or in a social setting?* and/or *Does the child have mood swings that make it difficult for him to control his emotions?* Medications can help to stabilize a child's mood, resulting in better functioning at home and at school.

- **Risk-Benefit Ratio**—*Do the benefits outweigh the risks?* Medications may help the child make better choices, focus more attention, or have more drive for success, however, every medication can have side effects. Encourage parents to educate themselves regarding different types of medications, including their uses, expected benefits, and side effects.

The goal of using medication is to help a child succeed, given the limitations caused by the TBI. If a child is successful while taking medication, he should receive the credit for his success. Similarly, if a child has a bad day while on medication, he should be held accountable for his behavior and receive appropriate consequences. His behavior should not be blamed on the failure of his medication.

Although medications can be effective and important components of treatment, they should not be viewed as a cure-all and typically do not eliminate the need for other forms of intervention, such as behavior management programs and counseling.

Return to School

A child's job is to go to school and learn. Returning to an educational environment is often the most important transition a child with TBI will have to make after leaving the hospital.

> Most gains in functioning after a TBI come from normal recovery, maturation, and growth; however, therapy regimens are important for safe and successful reintegration into home, school, and community life.

In the hospital, doctors, therapists, and staff are familiar with the effects of TBI and continually make accommodations for the child. In a school environment, however, it is unusual for teachers to work with a child who has a brain injury. Helping school personnel understand the child's strengths and weaknesses is critical in assisting them to develop appropriate accommodations and resource services for the child.

The following suggestions will help facilitate the transition of a child with TBI from a hospital or home setting to an educational environment appropriate to the child's functioning.

- Meet with the child's teacher to discuss the child's strengths and weaknesses. Describe the child's abilities and explain what is needed to help him succeed at school. Provide a list of classroom strategies (e.g., teach using a multi-modal approach) that are beneficial for the child.

- It is important to make sure there is a group of friends who understand the child's condition and can look out for him once he returns to school. Suggest that the child's friends visit him at home before he returns to school. You might also lead the friends in a discussion about the child's injury (with the child's and his parents' permission).

- Show classmates how they can help the child (e.g., arrange a buddy system for the child).

- Consider a half-day program when the child initially returns to school. Build up to a full-day program as the child can tolerate longer days.

- Work with the school to schedule difficult classes at times when the child is at his best (usually in the morning). Schedule easier classes in the afternoon when the child is likely to be fatigued.

- Share relevant medical reports and information with the child's school (with the parent's permission).

▌ Driving Following Brain Injury

For most adolescents, obtaining a driver's license is a high priority. The adolescent's independence, self-esteem, and employment opportunities are often dependent on the autonomy that comes from being able to drive.

For many parents, allowing their teenager to get behind the wheel can be a nerve-wracking experience due to the inherent dangers adolescents face while learning to drive. Parents of a teenager who had a TBI often have even greater anxiety. Their apprehension is compounded by the fact that most TBIs result from motor vehicle accidents and their child has a very real risk of sustaining a second injury.

Parents need to consider multiple factors when determining if their teenager is ready to drive following a brain injury. It is less important to determine if he can physically operate a vehicle and more important to determine if he has the cognitive capacity to deal with the complex situations he will face when he is behind the wheel.

The American Medical Association (AMA) holds physicians ethically responsible for notifying the state's Department of Motor Vehicles (DMV) when a patient has re-occurring seizures, loss of consciousness due to a TBI, or a compromised ability to safely operate a vehicle. Thus, physicians routinely report patients who have sustained a brain injury to the DMV. The DMV then suspends the patient's license or license eligibility until he is medically cleared to drive. The state may require the patient to have a driving evaluation and/or take a driving course before he can obtain a permit or license. Sometimes the patient may also need a physician's prescription in order to be referred to the driver evaluation center.

Factors that Affect Driving		
Physical Factors	**Cognitive Factors**	**Emotional Difficulties**

■ Vision (e.g., accuracy and speed of eye movements, peripheral vision, visual neglect)
■ Hearing (e.g., acuity or inability to recognize sounds [*auditory agnosia*])
■ Physical/Motor Ability (accuracy, coordination, speed, and reaction time)
■ Sensory Loss (can disrupt accuracy and strength of movements)
	■ Attention
	  • ability to focus for a prolonged period
	  • ability to filter out external and internal (daydreaming) distractions
	  • ability to process and manipulate information mentally
	■ Executive Functioning
	  • speed of information processing
	  • ability to multitask and rapidly switch attentional focus
	  • flexibility of thought
	■ Problem Solving
	■ Judgment
	■ Visual-Spatial and Visual-Perceptual Abilities
		■ Anxiety
		■ Depression
		■ Risk-Taking Behaviors
		■ Aggressive Behaviors
		■ Impulsivity
		■ Disinhibition
		■ Frustration Tolerance
		■ Emotional Lability and Control

▌ Transition to Adulthood

The transition from adolescence to adulthood will be easier for an individual with a disability when parents and professionals are prepared. They need to make decisions involving education, vocational options, guardianship, conservatorship, financial decisions, and insurance benefits before the adolescent becomes a legal adult. Planning for the future may include the following considerations.

- Educational services change from public school services to state departments of vocational rehabilitation services, adult educational programs, or disabled student services in college.

- Only the courts (i.e., probate or family) can legally determine if a person is incompetent or incapacitated due to cognitive impairment and if he requires a legal guardian. Guardians should be appointed before the adolescent turns 18.

- Financial assets and benefits may require management by a conservator (guardian of person and/or property).

- Health insurance companies should be notified of the adolescent's disability and need for continued coverage. Medicaid and/or Medicare may be an option. Information regarding eligibility is available from the local Social Security office.

- Young adults with mental disabilities are at high risk for being victimized financially when they become "legal adults." They may become victims of sales schemes, fraud, and even supposed friends who take their valuables or money.

- Various housing options may need to be considered (i.e., independent living, college dorm living, supervised residential placement, etc.).

▶ **Audiologist (AuD, CCC-A)** — An audiologist specializes in identification and assessment of hearing loss and other auditory, balance, and related sensory-neural problems. Audiologists also assist with the management of symptoms and rehabilitation for such problems.

▶ **Child Life Specialist (CCLS)** — Child life specialists are professionals who help children and their families cope with challenging life situations and stressful hospital experiences. Child life specialists provide developmental, educational, and therapeutic interventions for children and their families. They also attempt to alleviate the stress and anxiety that many children experience as a result of being hospitalized or experiencing a chronic illness.

▶ **Dietitian (RD)** — A dietitian is a professional who specializes in the nutritional needs of a brain-injured patient. Nutritional needs can change after a brain injury and feeding may be difficult due to medical complications, such as a tracheotomy, oral-motor apraxia, facial bone injuries, gastrointestinal injury, etc. The use of feeding tubes is also monitored by a dietitian.

▶ **Family** — Family caregivers are very important members of a treatment team. Family members and caregivers provide encouragement, assist with activities of daily living, supervise and protect the child, provide ongoing therapy and educational stimulation, and provide emotional security and comfort during a difficult time in the child's life.

▶ **Neurologist (MD, DO)** — A neurologist is a medical doctor who specializes in disorders relating to the central nervous system (brain and spinal cord) in addition to peripheral nerves. Neurologists are important in treating medical complications such as seizures, peripheral nerve problems, spasticity, headaches, etc.

▶ **Neuropsychologist (PhD, PsyD)** — A neuropsychologist is a doctor who specializes in brain functioning and how normal and abnormal functioning of the brain affects cognition (thinking, language, memory, visual-spatial processing, etc.) and motor and sensory functioning. Neuropsychologists assess brain function and identify brain-related disabilities or limitations that may affect functioning. The identification of cognitive strengths and weaknesses is important in developing a treatment plan for a child. Neuropsychologists may also provide therapy designed to improve brain functioning relating to cognition.

▶ **Neurosurgeon (MD, DO)** — A neurosurgeon is a medical doctor who is a surgeon specializing in disorders of the central nervous systems (brain and spinal cord). Neurosurgeons are important in treating medical complications such as increased intracranial pressure, bleeding in the brain, skull fractures, spinal cord injuries, etc.

▶ **Nurse (RN, LVN, PNP)** — A nurse is a medical professional who, under the guidance of a physician, assists in the care of a patient. Nurses deal with the day-to-day treatment of a child and perform such duties as assessing vital signs, level of alertness, nutritional needs, hygiene needs, bowel and bladder programs, etc. In addition, they administer medications as dictated by a physician. Nurses are also important in helping a brain-injured child to get out of bed and dressed so that he can start therapy, or in providing information about the child's functioning.

▶ **Occupational Therapist (OTR)** — An occupational therapist is a professional who specializes in the motor, cognitive, and perceptual functions that allow a patient to perform the many things that occupy his life (activities of daily living). Occupational therapists may work on dressing, hygiene needs, play behaviors, physical aspects of education (writing, drawing, visual-spatial processing), and work-related needs, such as typing. They may also work with other members of the team on feeding and swallowing problems. Occupational therapists also assess for the appropriateness of adaptive technology and help a patient use it to increase his functioning.

▶ **Patient Care Technician (PCT)** — A patient care technician is a professional who assists patients with many tasks that the patients are unable to do for themselves while they are in the hospital. Patient care technicians help the patients with activities of daily living, such as eating, getting out of bed, brushing their teeth, combing their hair, and bathing. They may also supervise the patients who cannot be left alone and require one-on-one supervision due to safety or medical reasons.

▶ **Physiatrist (MD, DO)** — A physiatrist is a medical doctor who specializes in physical disorders involving the body and limbs, and rehabilitation that may or may not include traumatic brain injuries. Physiatrists are important in treating medical complications such as spasticity, loss of limb function, etc., and have expertise in the use of prosthetic and assistive devices used to maximize functioning.

▶ **Physical Therapist (MPT)** — A physical therapist is a professional who specializes in the physical functioning of a person as it relates to movement. Physical therapists assess and provide therapy relating to the large muscle systems of the body responsible for walking, trunk control, sitting, transferring in and out of a wheelchair, and other activities necessary for activities of daily living. They also deal with range of muscle movement, endurance, motor planning, and use of adaptive equipment, such as orthotics, wheelchairs, walkers, etc.

▶ **Psychiatrist (MD, DO)** — A psychiatrist is a medical doctor who specializes in emotional and behavioral aspects of a patient's functioning. Psychiatrists assess for emotional and behavioral disorders and develop a treatment plan that may include medications, therapy, or a combination of the two.

▶ **Psychologist (PhD, PsyD)** — A psychologist is a doctor who specializes in the emotional and behavioral aspects of a patient's functioning. Psychologists focus on assessment of emotional disorders and providing therapy to help a child adjust to his new deficits. They also provide assistance in controlling a child's behavior after a brain injury by recommending behavioral modification programs to be implemented by other members of the team, including family members, nurses, therapists, etc.

▶ **Rehabilitation Counselor/Vocational Therapist (CRC)** — A rehabilitation counselor or vocational therapist is a professional who assesses a patient's academic and work-related skills in order to assist him with return to school or the workplace. They also educate disabled individuals about their rights under state and federal laws (e.g., ADA) and various governmental resources available to the patient relating to training, equipment, and vocational placement.

▶ **Respiratory Therapist (RRT)** — A respiratory therapist is a professional who specializes in a patient's respiratory functioning. Respiratory therapists monitor and adjust tracheotomy and ventilator functioning. They assess and provide treatments relating to breathing. They work closely with the nurses and pulmonologists, who are medical doctors that deal with lung and breathing problems.

▶ **Social Worker (MSW, LCSW, MFC)** — A social worker is a professional who serves as a link among the patient, family, and social service agencies or other community resources. Social workers assist with financial issues and patient needs after discharge. Social workers also often provide therapeutic counsel to families and caregivers and act as their advocate.

▶ **Speech-Language Pathologist (MA, CCC-SLP)** — A speech-language pathologist is a professional who specializes in language- and communication-based disorders. Speech-language pathologists assess limitations involving language and nonverbal communication. They also assess oral-motor functioning relating to speech, eating, drinking, and swallowing. Speech-language pathologists provide therapy designed to improve communicative functioning and oral-motor abilities. They evaluate for the appropriateness of augmentative communication devices and provide therapy designed to help a person use such devices.

▶ **Therapeutic Recreation Specialist (CTRS)** — A therapeutic recreation specialist is a professional who provides a child with a brain injury the opportunity to participate in leisure activities. Therapeutic recreation specialists are helpful in identifying and adapting activities so that a child can participate in them. Therapy is generally done as a group activity, with several children interacting in a play environment. The therapeutic recreation specialist works with other members of the team to develop leisure activities that are both fun and therapeutic for the child.

Chapter 10

Intervention

Intervention means different things at different stages of brain injury recovery.

- In the emergency department, intervention means stabilizing the child's medical condition to preserve life.

- In the pediatric intensive care unit (PICU), intervention is focused on bodily functions that are necessary for sustaining life. For example, attention is directed to respiratory function, intracranial and systemic blood pressure, metabolic activity, and the organs that may have been injured in the accident, such as the kidneys, spleen, and liver.

- In the medical rehabilitation unit, intervention is focused on the child's functional needs, such as getting him to sit, eat, walk, or move around the room. Cognitive intervention involves working on language and mental functions required for normal activities of daily living. The focus of therapy involves safety awareness, judgment, insight into deficits and strengths, and the ability to communicate needs. Children also receive assistance in their day-to-day functioning, such as setting realistic goals, following a therapy schedule, and adapting to their deficits.

- After discharge, intervention focuses on social participation involving school and play and for older adolescents, employment. As the child matures and shows improvement in safety awareness and judgment, the focus shifts to independence.

This chapter covers important intervention issues relevant during the medical rehabilitation stage of recovery. The goals of rehabilitative therapy include maximizing outcomes and facilitating cognitive recovery. Those involved with the child's care should continually monitor cognitive and communication functioning because changes occur fairly rapidly during this stage of recovery. Treatment goals should be realistic to the patient's needs and his developmental, social, and cultural environment.

Short-term goals should focus on improving cognitive functioning.

- increased awareness of the environment (lower-functioning children)

- increased ability to interact with surroundings (lower-functioning children)

- increased ability to reason and problem-solve or to do academic tasks (higher-functioning children)

- improved verbal and nonverbal communication skills (higher-functioning children)

Long-term goals should involve functional activities and transitioning.

- increased ability to participate more fully in activities of daily living (ADLs), such as dressing, brushing teeth, and eating

- improved judgment and safety awareness

- transitioning from the highly-structured hospital environment to a less-structured home or school setting

- return to a previous job or establish gainful employment (for an adolescent who has completed his formal education)

An additional goal of therapy is to find ways to increase a child's tolerance for therapeutic intervention. Therapists can increase a child's participation in therapy by making it fun, doing things that interest the child, and involving family and friends as appropriate. Often, having a child work with a brother or sister can facilitate participation and cooperation. The use of therapy dogs can also help motivate a child and facilitate participation.

The rate of recovery varies for each child. By being observant and creative, you will be able to develop a number of strategies specifically tailored to the needs of the individual child. You should reassess the strategies frequently so you can fade out strategies that are no longer appropriate and add new ones as necessary to meet the child's changing needs and interests.

▌ Choosing Therapy Activities

> Spice up your therapy sessions with **PEPPER**.
> - **P**rovide multiple opportunities for therapy throughout the day.
> - **E**ncourage and expect participation.
> - **P**ractice frequently and at times when the child is alert.
> - **P**rovide reinforcement.
> - **E**ngage the child with whatever is interesting to him.
> - **R**epeat tasks to facilitate overlearning of new skills and incorporate prior learning.

When choosing activities, keep in mind that brain injuries can cause perceptual and/or movement problems which may interfere with therapy. Perceptual problems can affect the child's awareness of visual, auditory, and tactile information. It is especially important to note if the child has difficulty with vision because he will often be unaware that he is not seeing some of the information. For example, a hemi- or quadranopia may be the reason he does not consistently identify objects or pictures correctly. (See Chapter 6, pages 105-111, for more information regarding visual impairments following brain injury.)

If a child has difficulty with an activity, simplify it. If the activity seems too easy for the child, make it more difficult. Creativity is important in therapeutic intervention because a child will be more likely to "stick with the program" if he views it as a fun game or activity. Over time, the activities themselves may become self-reinforcing and can be used as rewards for completion of more challenging tasks.

Case Example 1 *John*

Dr. Lebby evaluated John, a 9-year-old, who was unable to integrate visual information with motor functioning due to his neurocognitive deficits. John was unable to write numbers or letters or draw basic shapes. The best way to train the developing brain to do these types of activities is through repeated practice, but John hated to draw because it was difficult and he felt "stupid" when he couldn't make the right shapes.

Dr. Lebby asked John what he liked to do, and John said he loved to watch car races with his father. Dr. Lebby drew a series of different "racetracks." He then gave one of the racetracks to John and asked him to draw a line that followed its course. John was to draw the line as fast as he could while Dr. Lebby timed him. Each time John went off the racetrack, he lost a second. If he went way off the track, he "crashed."

The game became a scored competition between John and Dr. Lebby. They each chose a driver's name and then raced repeatedly, using many different tracks just like in NASCAR. John enjoyed "racing" so much that Dr. Lebby used the races as a reward for John when he worked on things that he disliked. Dr. Lebby transformed a task that John refused to do into a task that was rewarding and fun. As a result, John's participation and cooperation improved dramatically.

Brain injuries often lead to inconsistencies in functioning—some skills are spared while others are impaired. Because of this, a child with a TBI may be able to do a difficult task but not an easy one. When a child has intact functioning in some areas, it is difficult for people to understand how he can have so much trouble in other areas. The child may also have retained some prior learning which may suggest that he is cognitively intact. This may lead others to believe that his cognitive impairment is not severe and that he is just being lazy or he is not trying hard enough. In addition, even though his prior learning may be mostly intact, a child with TBI commonly has impairments in his ability to learn new information.

A child who has sustained a TBI often requires assistance to function optimally following discharge from the hospital.

- The child may need modified schoolwork.

- The child may need extra time to get ready for school or complete assignments and chores.

- The child may require assistance to help him focus on relevant information (e.g., cue him to focus on a task, point out the next problem on a worksheet, etc.).

- If the child has motor deficits, he may need someone to take notes or help him move from one classroom to another.

- If the child has motor deficits, he may need assistance to complete chores, such as clearing the dishes, folding laundry, or taking out the garbage.

174

- Fatigue is often a big problem after a TBI, so the child may need frequent breaks during the day or a shortened school day. A child who did not previously require naps may need downtime during weekend activities or at the end of a lengthy school day.

Feeding and Swallowing

It is common for a child to lack adequate, nutritious intake and/or have difficulty swallowing following a brain injury. Therefore, every child who is referred for a speech-language assessment should be given a bedside swallow evaluation.

> Poor food intake can be due to a variety of factors:
> - medical complications
> - coma or reduced arousal
> - dysphagia
> - cranial nerve damage or disruption
> - lack of appetite

It is the speech-language pathologist's and attending physician's responsibility to evaluate the child's ability to swallow safely when he is ready to take foods by mouth. Poor swallow reflexes can result in food passing into the trachea or lungs instead of the esophagus and stomach, a condition that can cause pneumonia and become life-threatening. When it is unsafe for the child to eat by mouth, nutrition should be provided by tube feeds (e.g., nasogastric tube—NG, gastrostomy tube—GT).

A child who fails the bedside evaluation or shows symptoms of oral-motor dysfunction may also require a *videofluorographic swallowing study* (VFSS) to evaluate his swallowing ability. The VFSS is usually performed jointly by an SLP and a radiologist or physiatrist. For this study, the child consumes foods and/or drinks mixed with barium to make them visible on an *X-ray*. As the child eats, X-ray-type images are observed on a video monitor and recorded for review by a radiologist.

The VFSS is similar to the *modified barium swallow* (MBS). The only differences are that small bolus volumes are used in the MBS, and the procedure does not include drinking from a cup. In clinical practice, the terms *videofluorographic swallowing study* and *modified barium swallow* are often used interchangeably.

Note: Further information regarding swallowing evaluation, therapy, and therapy goals are outside the scope of this text. For more information, we direct you to other resources regarding the mechanisms of swallowing, evaluation of those mechanisms, and therapeutic interventions for such conditions.

Intervention with Children Who Have Neurological and Cognitive Deficiencies

The following sections provide some general information regarding issues related to neurological and cognitive deficiencies and limitations resulting from a brain injury. Goals and intervention activities are included for use as appropriate, given the child's age, developmental level, general level of functioning, and physical abilities. Appendix 10A, page 202, provides information regarding strategies that may facilitate appropriate communicative interaction with patients and families.

Receptive Language

Receptive language deficits often result in the child misunderstanding instructions and task requirements. To remediate receptive language difficulties, use both verbal and visual modes of presentation for instructional techniques. Often, only a verbal mode of presentation is used for novel information and directives at home or in the classroom. Utilization of a multimodal (verbal and visual) means of presentation, however, may improve the child's comprehension and conceptualization of the material.

Accommodations to Improve Receptive Language

- Give instructions in simple, concrete, and understandable terms. The instructions should be appropriate, given the child's cognitive and language proficiency.

- Have the child repeat back instructions to confirm that he was paying attention and understood the information.

- Watch for signs of confusion and frustration (e.g., puzzled looks, crying, anger outbursts, withdrawal, attention deficits). These signs may indicate that the child is having difficulty understanding what you are saying.

- Include many modes of communication, such as pictures and written words.

- Break down information into single, understandable units (e.g., give one direction at a time) to assist the child in overcoming limitations. Ensure that the child comprehends each unit before moving on to the next component.

- Slow down your rate of speech and use simple, positively-phrased sentences.

- Do not use slang or unusual forms of speech.

- Avoid using complex language concepts, such as innuendo, metaphor, or analogies.

- Reduce or eliminate environmental sounds or noises whenever possible, as they may be distracting.

- Use gestures appropriately in conversation (e.g., hand gestures, facial expressions, body movements).

- Face the child and make eye contact so he can utilize visual cues from your facial expressions.

- Use information that is familiar and relevant to the child to introduce new ideas.

- Repeat words or phrases that can be misheard (e.g., *14* for *40*, *Bill* for *Phil*).

- Check frequently to ensure that the child is completing the task correctly.

◆ **Low-Level Goal:** *The child will follow simple, one-step directives.*

It is necessary for a child to follow simple directions so he can safely participate in activities of daily living. First decide which directive you want to teach (e.g., *Stop, More, Point to the _____,* or *Give/Get me the _____*).

Activity 1: Place one or more color photographs in front of the child. Choose the number of photographs to use based on the child's attention, comprehension, and discrimination skills. Then say, "Point to the _____." Note: You may use drawings, but it is usually easier for the child to identify color photographs.

Activity 2: Place one or more objects in front of the child, depending on his level of functioning. The objects should be common, relevant, and familiar to the child (e.g., for young children—a ball, toy car, or a cup; for older children—keys or a cell phone). Say, "Give me the _____."

Activity 3: If the child is ambulatory (walks, runs, or uses a wheelchair independently), you may choose to teach him to respond to *stop*. Have him play with toy vehicles. Teach him to stop the vehicle when you give a verbal command or show the nonverbal "red light" cue card.

If the child does not stop when you ask him to, physically assist him in stopping the vehicle for a short period. Then say, "Go" or show the child the "green light" cue card. Once a child has demonstrated a consistent ability to follow these directions with toys, generalize the skill to a variety of other physical activities. Activities in the child's room, in a gym, or on the playground can be utilized to further teach the child to stop physical movement on command.

Activity 4: For a child who is severely aphasic, begin by working on nonverbal sounds. Show the child three pictures (e.g., a cat, a duck, and a bus). Say, "Point to the picture that matches the sound I make." Then make a sound associated with one of the pictures (e.g., "Meow," "Quack," "Vroom-vroom"). Eventually say the name of the object and the sound together (e.g., "Cat says meow"). After some practice, the child should be able to point to a picture when you say the animal's name.

◆ **Moderate- to High-Level Goal:** *The child will follow multi-part directions.*

The child will be expected to follow multi-step directions once he leaves the hospital and returns to school or a vocational environment.

Activity 1: Have the child follow a series of directions that require him to build a structure with Lego blocks or tubing. As the child improves, use more complex directions and designs. Example: *Use eight yellow blocks to build a tower. Then put a blue block on top of the tower and a red block beside the tower.*

Activity 2: Develop some sample classroom assignments to use with the child. Help the child break down the task into smaller steps by identifying each one. Then help him write a list of things he needs to do to complete the assignment. Example: *Put your name on the top of your paper. Complete items 1–10 on page 15 and items 25–30 on page 16. This assignment is due on Wednesday. It should be turned in with your homework at the beginning of class.*

Activity 3: Use a phone book as a therapy tool. Tell the older child/adolescent that you need a new TV. Then have him look in the phone book to find a place where you could buy one. To make the task more complicated, give specific details that the child needs to understand in order to achieve the task. Example: *I would like to buy a new TV, but I do not want to buy it from a department store. I would like to have it delivered this Saturday.*

Expressive Language

It is common for a child with TBI to have word-finding and verbal formulation difficulties. When a child's speech is limited, start by working at the child's level. Do not overwhelm him with a lot of details. If you reduce your expectations for the child to respond in great length or detail, he may be more inclined to open up and attempt to respond to simple questions or join a conversation.

Accommodations to Improve Expressive Language

- Cue the child to let him know when he is going off topic.

- Ask the child *wh-* questions to get him back on topic.

- Ask the child questions that provide a choice to determine if he knows an answer to a question. Because the child's language deficits may interfere with his ability to talk about a topic, his verbal responses may not accurately reflect his knowledge. He may know more than he is able to communicate.

- Allow extra time for the child to initiate a response when he exhibits verbal formulation difficulties, slowed processing speed, or long latencies.

- Provide assistance with vocabulary when the child has word-finding difficulties. Say the correct word, a more appropriate word, or a phonemic/semantic cue.

- If a child has fluent aphasia or logorrhea, use a visual, tactile, or verbal cue to indicate that a pause in communication is needed.

- Use materials that are colorful, familiar, meaningful, and desirable to the child.

- Choose topics that are interesting to the child and fit his life experiences.

Accommodations to Improve Expressive Language, *continued*

- Do not use abstract language concepts, such as metaphor, sarcasm, or analogies, as they may be difficult for the child to interpret.

- If a child produces a paraphasic or neologistic error, correct him and continue your discussion. If the child produces many paraphasic or neologistic errors, it may be helpful to ignore the errors. Continually correcting the child's speech can result in frustration and is disruptive to the conversation. These errors often resolve on their own with time and continued recovery.

◆ **Low-Level Goal:** *The child will increase his ability to attend to the environment and engage in communication.*

Activity 1: Use musical instruments to gain the child's attention and interest. Take turns playing an instrument with the child. Encourage him to request to take his turn using hand signs, vocalizations, or words.

Activity 2: Sing familiar songs, such as "Itsy Bitsy Spider" or "Old MacDonald." Encourage the child to sing with you because the familiar lyrics may facilitate increased expressive language skills. After a while, stop near the end of a phrase, leaving off the final word. Allow the child to fill in the missing word. After some practice, the child may be able to fill in two or more words.

Note: It is not uncommon for a child with a TBI to start singing or humming to a song before speech returns. In these children, the language areas may be more damaged than the areas that process intonation, melody, and other nonverbal aspects of speech. We have heard many children with aphasia vocalize to songs but not be able to produce verbalizations spontaneously or through imitation.

Activity 3: Engage a child (or a small group of children) in a conversation about a topic that is interesting to him and relevant to his life. For example, prior to a field trip, have the child discuss what he might see. After a field trip, have the child tell someone else what he did and saw. Use a cue, such as a hand signal, cue card, or key word, to let the child know when he is going off topic. You can also ask the child *wh-* questions to get him back on topic.

◆ **Low-Level Goal:** *The child will request a pleasurable activity.*

Following a severe TBI, children may not have the ability to meaningfully interact with their environment or communicate with others. Teaching the child to request will help him develop environmental awareness and basic communication skills.

Activity 1: Use a toy that has lights and sounds to increase the child's arousal and encourage interaction. For children with motor or visual impairments, toys with large buttons that require little pressure work best. Dim the room lights to increase the toy's effect and to help the child focus his attention on the toy. Have the child press the button to turn on the toy. (If he needs help, use a hand-over-hand approach to assist him.) Let the toy run for a short time before you turn it off. Repeat this process several times. Then introduce a hand sign or sound the child must make to communicate that he would like to reactivate the toy. When the child uses the cue, activate the toy or allow it to run for a short time as a reward for his communication.

Activity 2: If the child has a severe oral-motor apraxia or Broca's-type expressive aphasia, print out photographs of activities he likes to do. Place several photographs in front of him and let him choose one. The child may point to the photograph or give it to you to communicate his desire. You can also print out photographs of family members, foods, and favorite objects to provide other choices for the child. Pictures of food, drinks, and a toilet can help him communicate when he is hungry, thirsty, or needs to use the bathroom.

◆ **Moderate-Level Goal:** *The child will increase his mean length of utterance (MLU).*

Activity 1: Read stories together and discuss what happens throughout the story. Ask *who, what, when, where, why*, and *how* questions about the story. If the child has difficulty answering open-ended questions, start by asking questions that provide choices. For example, *Did the boy live on a farm or in the city?*

Activity 2: Before this activity, ask the child's parents or teachers what he is currently studying in school. Then ask the child open-ended questions, such as *What did you do in science class this morning?* If the child is unable to respond to this type of question, cue him by asking, "Did you study gravity or temperature?" Encourage the child to respond appropriately to the question. If the child attempts to communicate using gestures or single words, encourage longer responses.

◆ **High-Level Goal:** *The child will improve his word-finding ability.*

Activity 1: Have the child name picture cards. Provide the first sound of the word (phonemic cueing) as needed to help the child retrieve the correct label.

Modify the task for the child with higher-level functioning by having him use more complex language to describe the relevant features of the object. For example, if the picture is of a car, you can ask the child "What is this?" (car), "What group/category does it belong to?" (vehicle), or "What is it used for?" (transportation). You can also have him use car in a sentence. As the child's word-finding ability increases, introduce synonyms and antonyms to continue building his vocabulary.

Activity 2: Play an association game with the child. Use common phrases, sentences, or nursery rhymes and leave out one word for the child to fill in (e.g., *salt and _____*, *mother and _____*, or *Jack and Jill went up the _____*). You can also make up sentences about the child for him to finish, such as *My name is _____*, *I like to play _____*, or *My favorite food is _____*.

Activity 3: Hide an object or picture from the child's view. Have the child ask *wh-* questions until he can gain enough information to guess the object you are hiding. Make a list of *wh-* questions to give the child an idea about the types of questions he can ask. Use general questions, such as *What category does the object belong to?* and *What do you do with it?*, as well as more specific questions, such as *What color is it?* or *What size is it?* Tell the child that he can ask any question he wants and that the list is just a guide. When the child correctly guesses the object, show the object to him. If the child is unsuccessful, show the object to him and demonstrate the task by giving examples of questions he could ask. Keep a tally card to see how many questions it takes for the child to guess the object.

You can also take turns guessing and keep a tally card for each player. After you each guess three objects, add up the number of questions each person asked. Whoever asked the fewest questions is the winner.

Speech Skills

Many children have spontaneous recovery of speech skills as they recover from brain injury; however, conditions such as paralysis, apraxia, or dysarthria may limit a child's recovery of speech skills or may result in unintelligible speech production. In these cases, therapy is required to help the child improve.

> A child who has been intubated may have hoarseness or stridor due to irritation of the vocal cords. Intubation can also stretch the vocal cords, making voicing difficult and quiet (low amplitude). Children with weak vocal cords sound like they are whispering. Typically, this does not require intervention and resolves spontaneously over a month or two. Rarely, a child may have vocal cord paralysis due to intubation. If the child's vocal quality or volume has not improved after a few months, he may need to be seen by a specialist, such as an Ear, Nose, and Throat doctor (ENT).

◆ **Low-Level Goal:** *The child will improve sound production.*

Activity 1: Using bubble wands, alternate blowing bubbles with the child. Often, children with apraxia have difficulty moving their mouth muscles to blow forcefully.

Activity 2: For children who have become mute due to severe apraxia or expressive aphasia, use a toy with a microphone and amplifier to work on imitation or repetition of speech sounds. (The authors use a toy robot with a microphone that can amplify the child's voice, record and play back the child's utterances, and light up when the child speaks.) Have the child imitate simple oral-motor actions, such as blowing or voicing into the microphone. The toy's sounds, lights, and/or movements will be reinforcing for the child. A regular microphone with an amplifier/ speaker system works well also. The child's efforts are reinforced when he hears his own sound production.

Activity 3: Use simple, sound-activated toys that move, light up, or play music. Have the child voice sounds to activate the toy.

◆ **Moderate- to High-Level Goal:** *The child will improve prosody, rate of speech, and intonation.*

Characteristics of speech, such as prosody, intonation, and rate, may be disrupted by brain injury—especially with injuries to the right hemisphere. Children with right hemisphere damage often speak in monotone. They sound the same whether they are happy, sad, telling a joke, or expressing a concern. Their speech is often slow and lacks variations in melody or rhythm.

Activity 1: Say a phrase using the appropriate rate and rhythm so the child can imitate you. Then have the child repeat the phrase while you time him. Let him know how long it took him to repeat the phrase. As the child improves, present longer statements by breaking them into sections and using a different rate of speech for each section.

Activity 2: Use poems, rhymes, or limericks to help the child learn how to modify his speech output. Have him imitate you and copy the rate and rhythm of your speech. Record the child and play back his attempts to help him identify when he succeeds in imitation and what he needs to do to improve his imitation. You may want to save the recordings so you can show the child how much he has improved over time.

Activity 3: Write a passage in a large-sized font and spread out the words on a sheet of paper. Have the child read each word as you point to it. Control the rate of the child's speech by changing the rate that you point to the words. This can give visual feedback to the child and can help when verbal and language-based skills are disrupted by brain damage.

Written Language and Visual-Motor Integration Skills

The ability to write following a brain injury can vary from the child having no difficulty with writing to the child being unable to hold a pen or pencil. Different brain injuries (i.e., the type of injury, location in the brain, and severity of damage) affect writing and drawing skills in a variety of ways.

- A child with hemiparesis may not have the necessary motor control of his hand and fingers to hold and use a writing instrument.

- A child with basal ganglia dysfunction may have a tremor that interferes with writing.

- A child's movements may be so slow that he cannot form letters or words.

- A child with ballism may experience sudden arm movements, such as swinging or jerking, when he tries to write.

- A child can lose the ability to write (*dysgraphia*) even though he does not have a problem with his motor functioning.

- A child may retain the ability to write but cannot integrate his visual information with his motor functioning.

Provide as many opportunities as possible for children to use visual-motor (eye-hand coordination) and fine-motor skills. These skills are important for writing and drawing, and children can improve their skills with practice. Free drawing, scribbling, coloring, and writing numbers and letters can help develop a child's visual-motor skills. Drawing, coloring, painting, playing with play dough or modeling clay, and manipulating small objects, such as paper clips, buttons, and coins, can help develop his fine-motor skills. It is important to consider the child's developmental stage when using small objects that can be mouthed or swallowed, or pose a choking risk. We strongly recommend assessment of risk prior to incorporating such activities, and close monitoring of the child during his use of small objects.

Accommodations for Visual-Spatial or Motor Limitations

- Reduce the length of written assignments. For example, if the assignment is to write sentences for all spelling words, allow the child to write sentences for only half of the words.

- Have the child write a portion of an assignment and complete the rest orally. Have another student, a teaching assistant, or an aide record the child's oral answers.

- Minimize the amount of copying. For example, if the assignment is to copy sentences and underline the subjects, allow the child to only write the subjects.

- Give the child more time to complete assignments.

- Have another student, a teaching assistant, or an aide copy homework assignments from the board for the child.

- Allow the child to dictate and submit assignments on tape rather than writing them.

- Have the child use graph paper or a sheet of lined paper for math problems. Using the columns and rows on the graph paper helps the child align his numbers, which may prevent confusion caused by poor penmanship. Lined paper turned sideways provides columns without the constriction of boxes for each number. This is helpful for the child who has difficulty writing numbers in small boxes.

- Allow the child to use a computer to complete class assignments and homework.

- Allow the child to tape-record lectures instead of taking notes in class.

◆ **Low-Level Goal:** *The child will improve directional control while holding a crayon, marker, or pencil.*

Activity 1: Take turns with the child making different strokes with a writing tool. Depending on the child's ability level, you may also have him color different shapes, draw a variety of shapes, or label shapes using simple block letters. Progress from easier items to more difficult items so that eventually the child can combine lines and circles to make shapes and letters. Circles are easiest, followed by vertical and horizontal lines, and then diagonal lines.

Activity 2: Have the child write numbers on paper or a dry-erase board. Encourage the child to practice counting out loud as he writes, or have the child draw his favorite object(s) or a simple scene. Engage the child in a discussion about his drawing to practice speech-language and organizational skills.

Activity 3: Use dot-to-dot worksheets to improve directional control. If published worksheets are too difficult for the child, make your own dot-to-dot drawings. They can be as simple as a large circle, a square, or a pentagon.

◆ **Moderate-Level Goal:** *The child will improve basic writing skills.*

Activity: Have the child practice writing the alphabet. Increase language skills during the activity by talking about each letter, naming a word that starts with that letter, and (if the child is capable) having the child describe a feature of the object.

◆ **High-Level Goal:** *The child will improve spelling and writing skills.*

Activity 1: Write words on index cards. Choose words based on the child's level of functioning. Show a word to the child. Have him study it carefully and say it out loud. Next have him close his eyes and visualize the word. Then turn over the index card so the child cannot see the word, and have him write the word. Have the child check his spelling by comparing his word to the word on the index card. Repeat the process if he spells the word incorrectly.

Activity 2: Provide the child with concrete instructions for the rules of spelling. (Note: Only use rules that apply consistently in spelling.) Reintroduce these rules periodically in order to promote retention and understanding.

Pragmatics

Social communication difficulties are frequently associated with TBIs. Many children with brain injuries, who have pragmatic deficits, may need to be retaught social skills that they took for granted prior to the injury. The effects of poor social communication skills can be frustrating for both the child and his family.

Accommodations for Social Communication Difficulties

- Structure the environment to support appropriate behavior and optimize on-task attention.

- Have the child participate in group conversations to practice appropriate social language, turn-taking, reciprocity, personal space, and boundaries.

- Have the child participate in role-play to learn/practice appropriate body language and the use of nonverbal cues.

- Have the child act as if he were another child in the class to assist him in taking the other person's perspective on a chosen topic.

- Work on one behavior or social skill at a time.

- Develop a cue that signals to the child that he is exhibiting an inappropriate behavior.

- Be a positive role model for the child. Model the skills you are trying to teach.

- Establish a reward system to reinforce the child's successes and appropriate behavior.

- Support the child's involvement in structured groups and activities.

- Provide encouragement and external motivators, such as rewards, to optimize participation and minimize apathy.

◆ **Low- to Moderate-Level Goal:** *The child will improve social pragmatics and the ability to relate with others in an appropriate manner.*

If you teach pragmatics in a one-on-one environment, the skills may not generalize to other environments or social situations. Therefore, it is helpful to use group therapy techniques when teaching pragmatics. Act as a mediator and social facilitator with a group of children to help them initiate and respond to each other appropriately.

Activity 1: Read a story with a group of children. Have each child write a question about the story on a small piece of paper. Put all of the questions in a hat. Have the children take turns picking a question out of the hat and answering it.

Activity 2: Play board games (e.g., *Candy Land, UNO*) that require turn taking, social interaction, and cooperation. Give each child a task to facilitate interaction and participation. For example, select one child to organize the game, another child to hand out the pieces or deal the cards, and a third child to collect the pieces and put the game back into its box. Rotate the roles. Monitor the children's social skills during the activity. Each time a child interacts, encourage him to use appropriate social language, such as *Please, Thank you,* and *Excuse me.*

Activity 3: Read a short story to a group of children, and then discuss the story with them. Present a problem that is related to the story. For example, if the story was about a train robbery, you might ask, "How could the detective find out who committed the robbery?" Have the children work as a team to come up with creative ways to solve the problem. You may also have two teams attempt to solve the problem separately and then compare their solutions.

For younger children, you can choose from many popular children's books, including *There's a Nightmare in My Closet* by Mercer Mayer, *Alexander and the Terrible, Horrible, No Good, Very Bad Day* by Judith Viorst, and *If You Give a Mouse a Cookie* by Laura Joffe Numeroff. We suggest that you allow adolescents to choose books on topics that interest them, as it can be difficult to engage them in conversation unless they are motivated to participate. You may have the group choose a topic by discussing interests, bringing favorite books to the group, or using a chapter from a classroom textbook. For an adolescent who has reading difficulties, ask his teacher or the school librarian to recommend books that are relevant to adolescents but are written at a lower reading level. You might also look for books at local teacher bookstores or check online booksellers.

Nonverbal Communication

Nonverbal communication, such as gestures, body language, eye contact, and facial expressions, conveys a lot of information during conversations. Lack of nonverbal skills, especially facial expressions, are common following a TBI. The child may not smile when he is happy, frown when he is sad, or furrow his brow and purse his lips when he is angry.

◆ **Low-Level Goal:** *The child will increase his use of a "social smile."*

Activity 1: For very young children, encourage an automatic smile by playing simple games, such as "Peek-a-boo." When the child produces an automatic smile, have him look at himself in a mirror as you talk to him about his smile. For older children, tell jokes or tease the child once in a while during your session. When the child responds with an automatic smile, reinforce the smile with social praise.

Activity 2: Make silly faces using a variety of facial expressions. Have the child imitate you to increase his awareness of his facial muscles and his ability to move these muscles.

◆ **Moderate- to High-Level Goal:** *The child will increase his ability to match facial expressions with his tone of voice.*

Note: You may need to teach the child facial expressions in a direct manner.

Activity 1: Have the child practice matching his facial expressions with his tone of voice through role-playing. The child can role-play a part in a script with the SLP, with his parents/siblings, or with a small group of other patients.

Activity 2: Have the child read dialogue from books and use facial expressions and vocal inflections to match the dialogue.

Activity 3: Have the child use appropriate facial expressions and vocal inflections as he imitates lines from movies (e.g., "I'll be back!" from *The Terminator*).

Emotion

Brain injuries can damage the parts of the brain that regulate emotional responses and behaviors. Children with TBI may show changes in emotion that range from flat affect to euphoria, and may have difficulty controlling their anger, impulsivity, emotions, and anxiety. Also, unlike a person with a developmental disability, a child with a brain injury functioned normally prior to his injury. Following the injury, memories of academic, social, and athletic successes can remind the child of his losses and reduce his self-esteem and confidence.

Because a child with TBI may experience a wide range of emotional, social, or behavioral difficulties, it is common for him to experience frustration and depression as he tries to adjust to his new cognitive and physical limitations. When a child shows signs of poor coping, counseling services should be readily available to assist him in adjusting to his limitations and to any associated emotional stress he may experience. Therefore, rather than offering specific goals, we recommend that you refer the child to a psychologist for an evaluation. A child psychologist or neuropsychologist experienced in working with children with brain injuries will be able to determine the nature and severity of any problem, as well as make appropriate treatment recommendations and goals.

> It is important for a child to work consistently with one psychologist. Good rapport and a strong bond with the professional are important so a child can feel comfortable voicing his concerns.

Vision

Visual Agnosia

Patients with visual agnosia have difficulty identifying objects by sight even though they can "see" without difficulty. Most patients with this condition can recognize an object by using their senses of touch, hearing, and smell. Since their reading skills often remain intact, patients can also recognize an object by reading its label.

◆ **Low-Level Goal:** *The child will improve the ability to identify objects.*

Activity 1: Use other intact senses to compensate for visual agnosia. For example, have the child handle an object, listen to the noise an object makes, or smell the object to help him identify it.

Activity 2: Have the child write labels for objects. Help him place each label on the correct object. Then have him figure out what each object is by reading the label.

Prosopagnosia

Patients with prosopagnosia have difficulty recognizing faces.

◆ **Low-Level Goal:** *The child will improve the ability to recognize faces.*

Activity 1: Have the child practice identifying photographs of familiar people.

Activity 2: Encourage the child to identify people and use names when gaining attention, asking questions, or conversing with others. It is also helpful to play games that require a player to ask another player a question. For example, when playing *Go Fish*, have the child use the person's name when asking for a card (e.g., "Randy, do you have a three?").

Visual Processing

Damage to brain areas around the primary visual cortex disrupts the ability to process complex visual information.

Accommodations for Visual Processing Deficits

- Have the child keep things organized without undue clutter.
- Teach the child where you keep things so he does not need to look in multiple places to find what he needs.
- Teach the child to slow down when navigating or looking for things.
- Use large pictures and/or fewer pictures per page on classroom handouts.
- Use a larger-sized font for written information.
- Keep the chalkboard/whiteboard clear of clutter. Only present necessary information.
- Keep the area well lit.

◆ **Low-Level Goal:** *The child will improve his visual processing skills.*

Activity: Have the child find hidden objects in complex pictures. You can find hidden picture pages in resources, such as *Highlights* magazine, and in books, such as *Where's Waldo?*

Visual Neglect

Patients with visual neglect fail to attend to one side of space. The failure to respond to and report stimuli on one side is not due to a vision problem but rather an attentional problem.

Accommodations for Visual Neglect Syndrome

- Always approach the child from his non-neglected side or talk to him as you enter the room to direct his attention so you do not surprise him.

- Sit on the non-neglected side to make it easier for the child to communicate with you.

- Turn the plate so the child will see and eat the food on the other side, if he neglects to eat food from one side of his plate.

◆ **General Goal:** *The child will improve his visual scanning skills to include the neglected side of space.*

Activity 1: Have the child play games in which he has to find stimuli, such as pieces of a puzzle, that are placed within his neglected field. Use brightly-colored objects or arrows that point to the neglected side to assist the child in directing his attention to the target stimuli. You may also incorporate verbal cues into this activity.

Activity 2: Have the child participate in a treasure hunt. Hide parts of the treasure in both the child's non-neglected field and his neglected side of space. Make the treasure hunt more interesting by having the child navigate around obstacles as he searches for the treasure.

Executive Functioning

TBIs usually result in executive function deficits involving attention, reasoning and problem solving, planning and organization, and sequencing. When the child has motor deficits or low energy, executive functioning difficulties can become worse. Accommodations should be provided for these difficulties in order to facilitate recovery and continued cognitive development.

Attention

Attention deficits that result from brain injuries are a neurological disorder and not a behavior disorder. A child's ability to attend to an activity is highly variable and depends on premorbid functioning and personality characteristics as well as the nature and severity of his brain injury.

Accommodations to Improve and Maximize Attention

- Use tasks that are interesting and relevant to the child.

- Give frequent and immediate reinforcement when the child pays attention to a task.

- Balance negative reinforcement with positive rewards. *Negative reinforcement* involves rewarding the child for completing a task by removing something he finds unpleasant (e.g., supervision). To make sure the child will work for positive reinforcements, you should not only provide negative reinforcement, but also supply positive reinforcement, such as giving the child something desirable once the task has been completed.

- Provide increased structure and consistency.

- Provide a private area or "distraction-free zone" for the child to do his work. Allow peers who do not have behavioral, attention, or academic difficulties to use the room, but only if they can sit quietly and work. If other children are not allowed to use the room, the child with attention problems may feel isolated or that he is being punished.

- Provide therapy individually or in small groups.

- Gain the child's attention prior to giving instructions.

- Frequently repeat instructions, especially during the early stages of recovery.

- Reduce the amount of work required, but keep the complexity and level of activities consistent with the work you give to peers. This adjustment will give the child with attention deficits more time to complete an activity and allow him to learn the same information as his classmates. It will also help to compensate for his poor focusing skills and lack of internal organization.

- Allow the child to stand next to his chair while working at his desk if he has difficulty remaining seated for any length of time.

- Engage the child in an activity that requires physical movement. He may have better attention when engaged in an active sport that does not require a lot of concentration or problem solving.

- Allow the child to participate in all recess and play activities (unless his behavior is aggressive or defiant of authority). It becomes increasingly difficult for children with attention difficulties, especially those with motor overflow (*hyperkinesis*), to remain seated and stay focused when they are not allowed to release some of their energy.

◆ **General Goal:** *The child will increase his length of sustained attention for a non-preferred activity.*

Activity 1: Have the child work on a scrapbook that requires cutting, writing, pasting, and organizing pictures and labels. Increase the period of time he works on the project each day/week.

Activity 2: Have the child maintain a journal or computer blog. Increase the length of time he works on the project daily/weekly.

Reasoning and Problem Solving

Children who have sustained a brain injury frequently have difficulty with a variety of reasoning and problem-solving tasks. If a child begins to show deficits in specific areas of functioning, provide accommodations and resource services in a timely manner to ensure that the child does not fall too far behind his peers, become discouraged, and/or lose confidence in his abilities. Adjust accommodations and resource services to match the child's age and functional abilities.

Accommodations to Improve Reasoning and Problem Solving

- Teach problem-solving skills directly (e.g., show the child the steps required to complete complex tasks, such as sequencing story cards or solving math problems).

- Assist the child in generating alternative solutions and strategies to solve a problem.

- Provide consistency and structure in the child's routine.

- Monitor the child's performance to ensure he is not falling behind his peers.

- Communicate all information and directions clearly.

- Use simple explanations and examples to clarify abstract concepts.

- Integrate new information with previously-learned concepts and knowledge.

- Simplify directions.

- Provide cues and prompts when the child has difficulty performing a complex task.

- Facilitate transitions from one task to another or from one mental process to another by providing cues and activity schedules/directions.

- Help the child check his work. Point out any errors he has made and help him correct them.

- Provide immediate reinforcement when the child completes a task or solves a problem.

◆ **Low-Level Goal:** *The child will develop the ability to generate multiple solutions when solving a problem.*

Activity 1: Have the child do basic symbolic matching tasks. Make two sets of three or four pictures. Begin with simple shapes and progress to pictures, such as a tree, a car, and a dog. (See Figure 10.1a.) Place one set down the left side of a whiteboard and the other set down the right side of the whiteboard in a different order. Ask the child to draw a line from one picture to its match. If necessary, demonstrate the task by drawing the first line across the page.

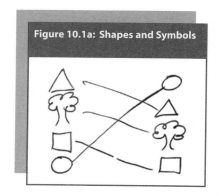

Figure 10.1a: Shapes and Symbols

In time, move on to letters, words, or numbers. Gradually combine numbers with squares to improve basic arithmetic awareness. (See Figure 10.1b.) The child will need to count the number of squares in order to find its match.

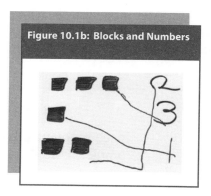

Figure 10.1b: Blocks and Numbers

Activity 2: Give the child a problem to solve. For example, you may say, "I need something to eat. What are some things I can do?" Help the child come up with solutions (e.g., go to the cafeteria, go to a restaurant, cook a meal at home, buy a snack at the store). Give reinforcement for each response to encourage the child to come up with more alternatives. Work with the child to help him decide which options are the best.

◆ **Moderate-Level Goal:** *The child will improve cognitive flexibility and language organization skills.*

Children with moderate brain injuries often think concretely because they lack the ability to process language information at the abstract or conceptual level. If you ask a child what a cow is, he may respond, "It has spots," or "It gives milk," instead of, "It is a farm animal."

Activity 1: Have the child sort picture cards into two categories (e.g., animals and food) to improve his language organization skills. As he sorts the pictures, have him name the item on each card and verbalize the appropriate category. When the child makes a mistake, cue a correct response by pointing to the appropriate pile.

Gradually increase the difficulty of the task as the child improves his sorting ability. You can either increase the number of categories or have the child sort the picture cards by subcategory (e.g., instead of food, have him sort by fruits, vegetables, and desserts).

Activity 2: Provide the child with two or more objects, pictures, or words. Ask the child to explain the similarities or differences between the items. Encourage flexible thinking by having the child give multiple responses to each set of items. For example, if the items are a house and a barn, the child could explain that they are both buildings, they are both places where people and/or animals live, and they are both found on a farm.

◆ **High-Level Goal:** *The child will improve problem-solving skills in real-life situations and environments.*

Activity 1: Have the child complete a real-life task that requires problem solving. For example, during therapeutic outings to a department store, give the child tasks, such as, *Find me something I can use to clean a spot from my carpet.* Provide cues and prompts as necessary to guide the child's progress.

You can develop similar tasks for the child who is in a hospital or a school. For example, have the child find something in the hospital's gift shop or find a specific book in a school library.

Activity 2: Have older children find information in the phone book. For example, tell the child you want to order a pizza. Ask him to find the name, number, and address of a nearby pizzeria.

Activity 3: Have adolescents fill out mock college or job applications.

Planning and Organization

TBIs can result in diminished planning and organizational skills. Children with TBI often lack initiation. They do not set goals for themselves and do not take steps to reach a goal once it is identified.

Children with TBI benefit from increased environmental structure and assistance with planning and organization. They may not, however, be aware of their cognitive problems and may fail to understand the need for external assistance or structure. Therefore, you should monitor them for difficulties and provide any necessary accommodations.

Accommodations to Improve Planning and Organization

- Establish consistent routines for the child's daily schedule.

- Structure the child's home and classroom environments with consistent rules.

- Physically organize the child's workplace.

Accommodations to Improve Planning and Organization, *continued*

- Provide structure for the child to complete activities of daily living (e.g., post a list of instructions on the bathroom mirror to help the child with his morning routine).

- Do not assume that the child will develop organizational skills independently. Provide direct instruction on organizational techniques (e.g., help the child organize his room using labeled boxes or drawers, teach the child to use an outline or graphic organizer prior to writing a report).

- Do not assume that skills taught in one subject area will generalize to another.

- Provide external prompts and structure to overcome complacency (e.g., Say to the child, "That was good. Now do the next one").

- Teach the child to request assistance with verbal cues, such as *I need help* or *Say it again*.

- Limit the amount of information presented in a task.

- Break down tasks or instructions into smaller steps. Give positive feedback as the child completes each step.

- Teach awareness of hindsight and foresight. Point out the child's previous mistakes and help him determine how to avoid the same mistakes in the future.

- Make a list of the steps the child needs to take to complete a task. Have the child check off each step as he completes it. Be aware that the child may stop in the middle of a task and require a prompt to finish it.

- Make a list of tasks the child needs to do during his morning and nightly routine and/or make a list of tasks to be completed during the day. Have the child check off each task as he completes it. Reward the child for checking the list, completing each task, and/or completing the entire list at the end of the day.

◆ **Low- to Moderate-Level Goal:** *The child will improve task completion.*

Activity 1: Have the child sort a deck of cards in different ways to reteach organizational skills. Begin by asking the child to sort the deck into two piles—black and red. If this is easy for the child, have him sort the cards by suit or by number sequence.

Activity 2: Play games with the child to teach skills such as planning ahead (foresight), developing strategies, and learning from mistakes (hindsight). Choose games like *Go Fish* for lower-functioning children and games such as *UNO*, *checkers*, or *Connect Four* for higher-functioning children.

Activity 3: Have the child describe the steps needed to complete a complex task. Write down the steps exactly as the child gives them. Then have the child attempt to complete the task by following his own instructions. Revise the steps as appropriate, helping the child identify the individual steps to complete the task successfully.

Sequencing

Children with brain injuries may be aware of the steps involved in a task, but they may do the steps out of sequence (e.g., putting shoes on before socks).

Accommodations to Facilitate Sequencing

- Outline the steps of a task for the child to follow. Place the outline in the area where the child will complete the task. For example, write the steps for using the computer on a sheet of paper and place the outline next to the computer. You can also write outlines on a dry-erase board which makes it easy to change the steps as the child improves.

- For children with verbal language disorders, outline the steps of a task using a series of pictures.

- Tape-record each step in routine activities, such as getting ready for school in the morning. Have the child listen to the tape in its entirety. Then have him listen to the tape again, pausing the tape after each step as the child works to complete the routine.

◆ **General Goal:** *The child will improve independent sequencing.*

Activity 1: Give the child step-by-step instructions for an activity, such as putting on his socks and shoes. Take photographs of the child as he performs each step. Then have the child complete the activity by following the sequence of pictured steps without your verbal instruction.

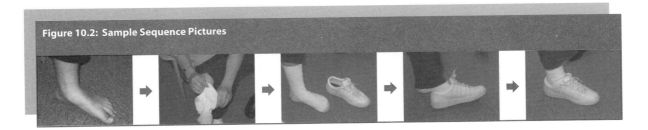

Figure 10.2: Sample Sequence Pictures

Activity 2: Have the child organize his activities for the day. Write the names of various activities that the child performs on cue cards. Have the child choose the activities he would like to do and then sequence them in the order he will perform them during the day. Placing the cue cards on a ring clip will help keep the cards in the correct order and make it easier for the child to carry them in his pocket or backpack.

Activity 3: Create cue cards that tell a story. Write one part of the story on each cue card. Then have the child arrange the cards in sequential order from the beginning to the end of the story. You can make this task easier by placing the cards in front of the child with one card out of order. Have the child identify which card is out of sequence, explain why, and then move the card to the correct spot.

Judgment and Behavior

Following a TBI, there may be a disassociation between a child's thoughts and his actions. The child may know right from wrong but may behave impulsively because he lacks the ability to self-monitor and regulate his behavior. He may also show impaired or diminished judgment which can lead him into dangerous situations.

TBIs may also result in increased irritability and a lowered tolerance for frustration. A child may become upset and exhibit outbursts of anger that are out of proportion to the situation. Following an outburst, the child may be sorry for his actions and show remorse. Outbursts may not be intentional on the part of the child; they are more often a function of the brain's lack of control over his emotions.

Accommodations for Behavior Issues

- Keep the environment relatively quiet by restricting the number of family members in the room.

- Turn down the lights and/or play soothing music to help the child tolerate therapy.

- Use behavior modification techniques that include consistent expectations and rewards for good behavior.

- Alternate between the types of tasks the child finds difficult and those tasks that are less affected by the injury. Going back and forth between difficult and easy tasks can prevent a child from becoming upset when he is having difficulty with a task.

- Watch the child for patterns that may indicate he is on the verge of losing his temper. Intervene by using relaxation techniques to help the child regain composure. For example, if a child becomes upset or angry during a task, stop the task and take a short break. During the break, help the child calm down by prompting him to think of pleasant things or by taking deep breaths.

Accommodations for Behavior Issues*, continued*

- Remind the child that he is doing well and not "failing." This can help him realize his gains and distract him from his ongoing deficits.

- Provide opportunities for the child to express his feelings.

- Help the child develop coping skills that are appropriate to various settings.

◆ **Low- to Moderate-Level Goal:** *The child will improve his ability to control tantrums and increase his frustration tolerance.*

Very young children or older children with severe impairments are not able to effectively regulate their behavior. Regulation must come from the environment and caregivers who know the child.

Activity 1: Expose the child to a less-structured environment and provide reinforcement for appropriate behavior. Also provide breaks during times when the child is unable to modulate his behavior appropriately.

Activity 2: During an outing or field trip to a store, give the child a task that requires interacting with the store's employees. For example, have the child ask a salesclerk to help him find a particular item. Cue appropriate behavior, politeness, manners, and social skills to facilitate the interaction.

Memory and Learning

Problems with memory are very common after a TBI due to damage involving the frontal and temporal areas. Memory deficits can be mild or severe enough to warrant a diagnosis of an amnestic syndrome (memory disorder). Therefore, it is important to understand the severity of the problem before beginning intervention with the child. This involves getting a history from the child's parent or caregiver and then interviewing the child to find out if past memories (premorbid) are intact.

Determine if the child knows the following:
- name
- date of birth
- age
- name of his school
- grade in school
- address
- phone number
- names of family and friends

You also need to determine if the child can recall recent events.
- Does he know where he is?
- Does he know what day it is?
- Does he know what activities he did today?
- Does he know what meals he ate today?
- Does he know the names of his nurses and therapists?

Although old learning may be intact, with the exception of the period close to the injury, new learning may be significantly disrupted. If the child has difficulties with new memories, you should inform his school personnel so that he can receive appropriate services and accommodations. When the child returns to school, he should be evaluated by school personnel to determine if he is eligible for assistance in the classroom. The type of accommodations will vary depending on the child's type of memory problem and the severity of the disorder.

Many times, memory problems do not completely resolve despite intensive therapy, practice, and repetition. Without accommodations at school, children with memory deficits will have significant difficulty learning new information. Additionally, without allowing accommodations during tests, you will simply be demonstrating that the child has a poor memory rather than evaluating the child's skills.

Accommodations for Memory Difficulties

- Provide a small teacher/student ratio.

- Reintroduce yourself each time you see the child, and have other staff do the same as often as necessary.

- Write the names of the child's doctors, nurses, therapists, etc. on a dry-erase board or on poster board in the child's room.

- Present information verbally as well as in written or picture format. This will help the child remember the information and allow him to review it as necessary.

- Design class assignments with extra structure. The child will be better able to organize his work and will reduce the amount of material that he forgets.

- Provide external memory devices, such as notebooks, diaries, day planners, and electronic schedulers.

- Keep the child's daily and weekly schedule as consistent as possible to minimize the amount of information he is required to remember.

- Allow the child to bring notes into tests or use other means to allow for optimal performance.

- Use "overlearning" techniques, such as frequent repetition, rehearsal, and review, to help compensate for memory limitations.

- Relate new learning material to something the child has already absorbed and mastered.

- Repeat task instructions. As children with TBI progress through school, instructions become more complex and more demands are placed on their memories.

- Give complex or lengthy instructions in a format that allows the child to refer back to the information. For example, write instructions on a whiteboard, have the child copy instructions into a "to do" book, or put the instructions on a handout. If the child has his own copy, he can cross off tasks as he completes them.

◆ **Low-Level Goal:** *The child will relearn his identifying information.*

Activity: Have the child print his identifying information on a wallet-sized card. Teach him to use the card when he is asked for this information.

◆ **Low- to Moderate-Level Goal:** *The child will use the names of people with whom he interacts frequently.*

Activity: Have the child write the names of the people he will be seeing on his daily schedule.

◆ **High-Level Goal:** *The child will improve his memory and independent ability to follow a daily schedule.*

Activity 1: Have the child record his daily schedule, important events, and other pertinent information in a "memory book." Include a calendar in the book. Each morning, have the child cross off the previous day and identify the current date.

Activity 2: Read stories that tell about sequences of events that are relevant to the child. Simple picture books that show children getting up, eating breakfast, going to school, playing, etc. may help reorient the child to basic daily routines. You may also use books, such as *Let's Go Froggy* by Jonathan London, *Elmo's Day* by Sesame Street, and *A Day in the Life of . . .* series by Dorling Kindersley Readers.

Activity 3: Have adolescents arrange sequencing cards (you can use cards with words or pictures). The activities may be simple routines performed throughout the day or a list of specific instructions to complete an activity. Choose routines/instructions that are meaningful to the adolescent and that will facilitate increased independence.

Visual Memory

Deficits in visual memory are common following TBI. Visual memory involves the following components.
- the ability to see objects
- the ability to identify the parts that make up an object
- the ability to remember the organization of objects in space relative to other objects
- the ability to recognize the objects' local and global characteristics

Memory and recall of visually-presented objects is a critical skill that is needed for much of the learning that takes place within and outside of school.

Accommodations for Visual-Memory Difficulties

- Provide the child with paper copies of pictures or charts that are presented during lectures (e.g., on an overhead projector).

- Verbally explain visually-presented information, such as pictures, charts, graphs, etc.

- Provide information in both written and visual formats to help the child utilize verbally-mediated reasoning to compensate for visually-based deficits.

◆ **Moderate-Level Goal:** *The child will recall details of objects presented to him immediately following the removal of the item and after a delay.*

Activity 1: Place an object or a photograph of an object on a desk. Let the child study the object for a short time. Then cover the object, and have the child try to recall its color, shape, size, etc.

Activity 2: Play "I Spy" with the child. Take turns giving clues and locating specific items.

Activity 3: Hide a few objects in the room while the child watches you. Later, ask the child where you hid the objects. Provide the child with clues as needed.

Activity 4: Have the child trace or free-draw visually-based information. For example, have the child draw a map of a state as you discuss facts relating to that state. Copying the information will help him learn and remember it.

Activity 5: Show the child a picture of an everyday scene for 15 seconds. Make sure the scene is not cluttered or complex. Take the picture away. Then ask the child questions about the picture, such as *What was under the bridge?* or *How many people were in the picture?*

Augmentative/Alternative Communication

Sometimes children never regain the ability to perform a task that is required for normal functioning. For example, some children may have relatively intact thinking ability but will never regain the ability to speak. Augmentative communication devices can help these children communicate.

We often use a notebook-sized computer with a touch screen. The computer displays pictures, phrases, words, letters, and/or numbers on the screen. The child can touch the screen to activate something that is displayed, and the computer will "speak" for him. Older children or adolescents can spell out sentences and have the computer "say" them. Another program allows the child to go to a "food" page and tap the screen over a picture of a hamburger or French fries. The computer then says something that corresponds to the choice, such as, "I would like a hamburger with fries, please." Other menus are available that deal with many different activities of daily living and communication needs.

Many augmentative/alternative communication devices are available. They can range from simple picture cards to very complex and expensive computers. We direct you to outside resources for further information regarding devices that may be beneficial for individuals needing sophisticated alternative communication modalities.

Academics

The Individuals with Disabilities Education Act (IDEA) is a federal law which mandates that schools provide special education services and/or accommodations to students who qualify because of special needs resulting from brain injuries. Once the school has determined that a child is eligible for special education services through the IDEA, the school is further mandated to develop an Individualized Education Plan (IEP) for the child in order to fully accommodate his unique needs.

> **The Individuals with Disabilities Education Act (IDEA), Public Law 101-476, Amended December 3, 2004: Public Law 108-446, Code of Federal Regulations (CFR) for Title 34**
> This act mandates that a person with TBI who qualifies for special education services must be provided with an appropriate education, regardless of the severity of his disability. Transition planning for work, community, and independent living after graduation also needs to be provided.
>
> **Americans with Disabilities Act (ADA), July 26, 1990**
> TBI is a recognized disability category under ADA. This act ensures that individuals with disabilities have access to all provisions of ADA and are accommodated in employment, transportation, government activities, and communication.

It is critical to evaluate a child with a TBI on a regular basis in order to determine any changes in functioning. The child may have deficient skills during one evaluation but may fall within normal limits a short time later due to continued brain recovery. Based on the results of your evaluations, you may find it necessary to suggest revisions to the child's IEP, including updated recommendations, accommodations, and therapeutic interventions as appropriate.

Use a performance-based grading system to compare the child's current level of functioning to his previous performance. Because this type of grading system is based on the child's own gains, any improvement he makes is an accomplishment, even if he is still performing below what is expected given his age or grade level. The child will perceive his own success and will not be continually reminded that he has impaired skills compared to his peers.

When a child with a TBI feels that he is succeeding and making improvements, he will gain confidence and self-esteem. He will also be more responsive to school and to additional tutoring because he believes that the extra efforts are helping him improve. (See Appendix 10B, page 203, for some general guidelines on facilitating school reintegration.)

Note: Be cautious about recommending treatment programs that are not evidence-based or that rely primarily on data from their own studies. There are many treatments available that show little or no gains above that expected from normal development, recovery, or placebo effects. Research programs and treatments before you suggest that parents enroll their child in a specific program. Look for double-blind, placebo-controlled studies in peer-reviewed journals, such as the *Journal of Developmental and Behavioral Pediatrics*, *American Journal of Speech-Language Pathology*, *Journal of Neuropsychology*, *Archives of Clinical Neuropsychology*, and *Pediatrics*. It is also important to keep in mind that when a treatment does not work, it may be best to try a different approach or reevaluate the clinical needs of the child.

Appendix 10A: Optimizing Communication

The following components are important when communicating with patients and families:

1. Be attentive and listen carefully.
2. Make every attempt to fully comprehend the intended message, without interrupting.
3. Communicate your understanding of the message to the patient and/or family.

Communication involves using and understanding nonverbal information. The use and identification of the following nonverbal cues may help you communicate with patients and families. You should also observe whether your patients effectively use nonverbal communication. If not, it may be helpful to formally address the use of effective nonverbal cues in therapy.

Eye contact — The speaker should look at the listener to hold the attention of the listener. If the speaker is looking at something else, the listener may be wondering what the speaker is looking at instead of attending to the conversation. The listener should also maintain eye contact so that the speaker knows that the listener is attending to the conversation. Staring-off usually indicates that the listener is thinking about something other than the conversation.

Facial expressions — Facial expressions should be relaxed, but also change appropriately with the topic. Flat affect usually indicates disinterest or a problem with the use of appropriate variations in facial expressions. Avoid grimaces, frowns, and irritated looks which are, at the very least, distracting and at the worst, detrimental to the conversation.

Nonverbal gestures — Many people use hand movements to facilitate communication. Subtle hand movements are best. Sudden or rapid hand movements are usually distracting.

Vocal tone/inflection — Vary the volume, speed, melody, rhythm, and inflection of speech so that your message can be accurately interpreted by the listener.

Body posture — The speaker should appear relaxed. He should lean slightly toward the listener and avoid fidgeting. Extraneous movements of the hands or feet can be distracting.

Personal space — It is sometimes difficult to judge how much space should be between the speaker and the listener. Too little or too much distance may cause the individuals to feel uncomfortable with the situation. Note if the person you are talking to moves away from you or attempts to move closer to you. Unless you know the person you are talking to or have good rapport with him, it is best not to physically touch him, although a pat on the hand, arm, or back is usually appropriate during emotionally difficult times. Communication also typically improves when there are no physical barriers (i.e., desks or tables) between the individuals.

Silence — It can be golden! Although it may feel uncomfortable at times, a pause in communication is okay. In fact, silence during a conversation can be used to facilitate communication. Families may be unsure about the complex information being communicated and may need time to think and formulate a response. Patients with slowed processing speed or language formulation difficulties also require more time during a conversation. If the speaker rushes the listener for a response, the listener may become anxious, feel pressured, and possibly stop participating in the conversation.

- Consider accommodations for test taking. Children with TBI may exhibit slowed processing speed, motor limitations, attention difficulties, and memory impairments. Given a child's individual strengths and weaknesses, some common accommodations you should consider include oral examinations rather than written examinations, multiple-choice formats, extra time to complete tests, and open-book/note tests.

- Avoid the use of timed tasks and tests (e.g., classroom tests, standardized achievement tests). Asking a child to hurry while completing a task may cause undue stress, frustration, or feelings of failure. Emphasize accuracy, persistence, and understanding of the material rather than speed or rapid recall of facts.

- Use frequent diagnostic testing to highlight pertinent strengths and weaknesses. Academic skills that may have been present before the child's injury may have been differentially affected and may recover at different rates. Allow for modifications of classroom accommodations and resource services as needed for each skill area.

- Reteach skills as often as necessary. Attention deficits may decrease a child's ability to perform tasks consistently. Just because the child can do a task one day does not mean that he will be able to do the same task another day.

- Do not mistake academic difficulties for behavior problems. When a child does not complete an assignment as instructed, you may believe that the child is being disobedient when, in fact, the child may not be able to complete the work due to cognitive limitations.

- Accentuate the positive. Do not be so concerned with the remediation of deficits that you forget to acknowledge the child's areas of strength. This is important because TBIs often result in decreased confidence and self-esteem, especially within an educational environment. To help the child build his self-esteem and confidence, encourage him to participate in fun, extracurricular activities that are areas of strength for him.

- Prepare homework and tests so that the child is expected to get approximately 80 percent of the questions correct. An 80 percent correct response rate has been shown to be the optimal success rate to encourage continued study while reducing frustration. When a child achieves performance levels greater than approximately 80 percent correct, it may indicate that the task is too easy for him. The child is not being appropriately challenged, which often results in reduced effort and complacency. If the child achieves performance levels lower than 80 percent correct, it may mean that the task is too difficult for him. The child may become frustrated and lose confidence, resulting in lowered self-esteem and, sometimes, behavioral outbursts.

- Check in with the child frequently to ensure that he is completing tasks appropriately. A child with communication deficits may not understand instructions regarding homework, may be confused about assignments, and/or may not know how to complete a task.

- Remember that each child is different and rates of recovery vary for each individual. By being observant and creative, you will be able to develop a number of additional strategies specifically tailored to the needs of the individual child. You will also be able to reassess, fade out modifications that are no longer necessary, and add new modifications to meet the child's changing needs.

Chapter 11

Family Issues

A brain injury to a child can be devastating to the family. When a child suffers a TBI, the child and his family may experience increased levels of stress, depression, guilt, fear, and/or sadness. Psychosocial distress can also cause impaired social skills and ultimately a disruption, or even loss of relationships. The adjustment to residual deficits and subsequent psychosocial problems can last for several years following the brain injury.

Rehabilitation programs that prepare the child and family for reintegration into the community can alleviate some of the distress. Educating family members about the child's strengths and weaknesses and arranging follow-up visits for troubleshooting problems that arise after discharge can help the entire family feel less anxious and more in control. Information that may help you to understand the challenges faced by persons with disabilities and ways to increase positive interactions is provided in Appendix 11A, pages 213-216. Additionally, therapy that targets improved communication among family members and reduced social isolation for the child can decrease frustration and help the family and child adjust to the child's condition.

When working with families, keep the following things in mind.

- Families should be active participants in the child's care. They should be involved in decision-making, determination of goals, and treatment planning. They should become valued members of the child's healthcare team.

- The family is the constant in the child's life, while treatment team members may change often. Be sensitive to the family's concerns and goals for their child.

- No family is ever prepared for a family member to have a brain injury.

- Each family has different financial resources, which range from being very limited to being able to afford private care.

- Each family member has different individual strengths and weaknesses.

- Family members often go through stages of grief. Although the child survived, the family grieves for what the child may have been and the loss of the life he would have had.

- Families go through a variety of emotions depending on the stage of recovery.

- Recognize that different families have different coping methods.

- Not all families can adequately cope with the added demands of a child with a brain injury.

- Not all family members are capable of learning how to care for a child with a brain injury.

- Respect the ethnic, racial, cultural, and socioeconomic diversity of families.

- Share information with the family regarding the child's goals and progress on a regular basis. Always speak in terms that the family can understand.

- Encourage the child and family to build a support network.

Emotional Reactions of a Child with TBI

Children with TBI may experience feelings that are incongruent with their situation or that may reflect how they view their condition. A child may express feelings that are out of character for him and are difficult for his parents to comprehend. It is important to understand that the child is not only experiencing a new situation, but also may have some ongoing confusion and memory disruption which further complicate his feelings.

Children with brain injuries may experience:
- a lack of control in many aspects of their lives
- low self-esteem and confidence due to their lack of independence
- feelings of failure due to their inability to fully participate in age-appropriate activities
- enmeshment with family members due to their dependency on them
- isolation from family, friends, and peers
- guilt about what others are sacrificing for them
- guilt for "causing problems" with siblings and/or parents
- guilt for taking all of the family's resources (e.g., energy, money, time)
- fear about the future

Emotional Reactions of Siblings

Siblings may experience feelings of fear, anger, and/or guilt. These are normal feelings that all children experience, however, they may be amplified for children who have brothers or sisters with a brain injury.

Fear

To help children cope with the fact that their sibling now has a brain injury, remind them of the following.

- No one can "catch" a brain injury.

- Being scared is a natural response.

- The sibling did not cause the injury. Younger children think about the world in an egocentric manner and may believe that their sibling was injured because of what they did or did not do.

- Just because the child with TBI may be irritable or aggressive, have emotional outbursts, or be unable to control his behavior, does not mean that he does not love his brothers and/or sisters or does not want to be with them. His emotional and behavioral difficulties are likely related to his brain injury and not to how he feels about his siblings.

- Difficulties with movement, poor attention, or ongoing pain may make it appear as though the child with the brain injury does not want to play with his siblings. Most often, however, the child avoids playing because it is too difficult to for him to participate, not because he does not want to interact with his siblings.

What Can You Do to Help Siblings Become Less Fearful?

- Help them feel in control.
- Explain what a brain injury is and what it is not (i.e., a disease). The more they know, the less likely they are to make up their own (often inaccurate) explanations.
- Teach them about their sibling's injury and what they can do to help him. Explain why it is difficult for their sibling to do the things he used to do.
- Help them decide what to tell their friends about their sibling's condition.
- Talk about what they should say at school.
- Help them gain more control of their situation and become active participants in the recovery process. Children are often scared because they do not know what to do. A little bit of responsibility (e.g., simply holding their brother's or sister's hand during therapy) can go a long way in reducing this fear.
- Seek professional counseling, if needed.

Anger

Children may feel angry about many things related to their sibling's brain injury, including:
- the amount of attention paid to the injured child
- the extra time and resources that go to the injured child
- different house rules for the injured child
- the additional toys and games that the injured child receives

Siblings may also become angry because they:
- blame the injured child for family problems
- cannot help their injured sibling
- have to deal with social issues at school (e.g., standing up for their sibling, dealing with ridicule and teasing, not having a "normal" life)

Guilt

Siblings may feel guilty because:
- they are healthy or uninjured
- they have conflicting emotions (e.g., they are angry with their injured sibling when they know they shouldn't be)

Emotional Reactions of Parents

Personality, life experiences, and understanding of the child's condition all play a role in how parents perceive and deal with their child's injury. Even though they may respond to their child's injury in different ways, most parents experience similar emotions.

Shock and/or Denial

Parents usually remain in a state of shock or denial while their child is in the emergency department or intensive care unit. They cannot believe what has happened and may have difficulty performing even simple daily functions. Often, parents fail to fully appreciate the severity of an injury. They may believe that it is "not that bad." Denial in the early stages of recovery is quite useful in giving the parents time to gain better control of their emotions before being confronted with the reality of the situation.

Anxiety

Parents may become anxious if they have a poor understanding of their child's condition, have limited information from doctors, or lack a clear prognosis. Difficulties relating to financial burdens, missing work, or simply finding the time to complete normal parental duties, such as picking up siblings from school, can also significantly increase anxiety for the parent of a child recovering from a TBI.

Guilt

Parents may feel guilty for not protecting their child well enough. They may also believe that they made poor decisions which endangered their child. In the majority of cases, the injury results from an unpredictable and unavoidable accident. If the injury could have been avoided, however, guilt can become overwhelming and quite disabling for a parent (e.g., a child was injured in a car accident because he was unrestrained instead of sitting in an approved safety seat).

Frustration

Parents generally feel helpless through most of their child's hospitalization. Because children recover from brain injuries slowly, parents also may feel frustrated at their child's apparent lack of notable progress on a daily or weekly basis.

Anger

When parents are tired, overwhelmed, scared, or feel out of control, they can become angry over the smallest issues. The authors often use the saying *It was the straw that broke the camel's back* when discussing parental anger outbursts. Most of the time, a small, relatively insignificant issue triggers an anger outburst. One father began to shout and express his frustration when his child was served the wrong side dish with his lunch. His anger seemed to be out of proportion to the mistake, especially when the issue was easily resolved by ordering the child a new lunch. The father's outburst was actually a manifestation of the emotional distress he had been experiencing since his child was injured. The lunch mistake simply pushed him over the edge.

How Can Parents Take Care of Themselves?

Parents need to understand that taking care of themselves is not a selfish act. Physically, they need to avoid things that wear them down (e.g., lack of sleep, poor diet, drinking). Parents who lack nutrition or sleep will not be at their best for the injured child. If parents take time out for themselves, the positive effects will benefit other family members, including the injured child.

As they move through the grieving process and are able to tolerate more information without becoming overwhelmed, parents can reduce anxiety and stress by seeking out as much information as possible about their child's injury. Parents should:

- ask the professionals to explain issues to them using vocabulary and language they understand
- have professionals write things down for them
- talk to others who have experienced the same situation
- get professional counseling for themselves or other family members, if necessary

Children often need a lot of help from their parents early in brain recovery, but parents need to realize that it is okay if they are not always with the child. The child may actually do better when the parents are not present during therapy. When the child works alone with a therapist, he is forced to attempt tasks more independently.

Changes to the Family Structure

It is natural to expect changes to the family structure after a TBI. Attention and resources will be drawn to the child with the brain injury and away from other family members. This situation may be temporary; however, the changes may be permanent if the child has permanent physical and/or cognitive disabilities.

Because of the inevitable changes to the family structure, it is important to maintain equality among siblings as much as possible. A little love and attention to all children in the family will go a long way to comfort them.

You can maintain fairness among siblings by avoiding:

- *differences in discipline*
  If the injured child shows inappropriate behavior, do not excuse it. It is important that he receives consequences for his actions, just like his siblings.

- *differences in attention*
  Set aside some special time to spend with the children who are not injured.

- *differences in family contributions*
  Expect the child with the brain injury to do chores he is capable of completing.

- *differences in gifts*
  If you give gifts to the injured child, reward his siblings with similar gifts to thank them for their support, help, and understanding.

- *differences in daily routines*
  If the injured child must take medications with breakfast, have his siblings take vitamins or other supplements at the same time so that he does not feel different.

How Does an Adult's Attitude Affect a Child with TBI?

> A child with a brain injury is a child first and a child with a brain injury second. Adults will find it easier to focus on what is normal about the child when they treat him just like any other child.

The expectations that an adult has for a child recovering from TBI will often dictate how the child feels about his injury. If an adult has low expectations for the child, acts as if the child is incapable of doing anything, or treats the child as disabled, the child will begin to function at a lower level consistent with those expectations (self-fulfilling prophecy). Reduced functioning resulting from low expectations is most common when the expectations come from those in a position of authority or respect, such as parents and teachers. If the child continually faces lowered expectations for functioning, he may eventually experience *learned helplessness*, in which he will believe that he has no control over the situation and will stop trying.

A child can transition from a state of learned helplessness and dependence to a state of independence with the assistance of those around him. When an adult has high expectations for a child, the child will perform better, regardless of his actual ability. The child will learn to recognize opportunities in which he can take control, cope more effectively, and excel. Dr. Lebby has used the term *learned hopefulness* for many years to describe the process by which a child learns about his positive attributes and abilities, and regains his confidence. A child can learn to be hopeful if he is encouraged to improve his functioning and participation in age-appropriate activities.

Children who feel good about themselves:
- are able to set goals
- are more willing to take reasonable and appropriate risks
- initiate interaction and participate in age-appropriate activities
- can acknowledge their strengths and weaknesses
- can make choices for themselves based on their likes and dislikes

To maximize the child's performance, your expectations need to be appropriate to his optimal abilities. A 70 percent to 80 percent correct response rate or level of achievement is usually optimal to maintain gains and future recovery/development. Thus, you should assign tasks that have a difficulty level which allows the child to achieve a success rate of approximately 70 to 80 percent.

- More difficult tasks that cause the child to have a lower success rate often result in frustration and decreased effort on the part of the child. Additionally, if a task is too difficult, the child has less opportunity to receive reinforcement for successful completion of the task. This situation reduces the child's incentive to dedicate a strong effort.

- Tasks that are too easy and allow the child to achieve a success rate above 80 percent often result in complacency and reduced effort on the part of the child. The child does not need to dedicate effort and attention to the task.

- Using appropriate goals and expectations will result in the child increasing his effort in order to succeed and receive reinforcement. When a child dedicates a lot of work and effort to a task, he is more likely to feel a sense of accomplishment and pride when he is successful. His successes then become self-reinforcing.

As the child improves in functioning, adjust his goals accordingly to allow for additional incentives and achievement of rewards through an appropriate degree of hard work and effort.

How Can a Parent's Comments Affect a Child with TBI?

Comments that parents make can be devastating to a child's confidence. This is especially true if conversations and interactions constantly revolve around the child's injury and deficits. If parents only focus on the child's deficits without paying attention to the child's strengths or praising his achievement and recovery, it is likely that the child will lose confidence and self-esteem. Confidence from a parent or caregiver can be the most powerful medicine for the child who is recovering from a brain injury. Those working with a child with a brain injury need to be therapists, educators, and most importantly, cheerleaders.

> Focus on the child's strengths and reward even the smallest achievements. If the child's deficits are always the focus of attention, the child will view himself as less capable.

Warning Signs Suggestive of Emotional Disorders in a Child

- Unusual Behaviors—Notice behaviors that seem out of character for the child. For example, if a child says, "I'm never going to school again," do not respond, "Yes, you are." Find out what is wrong and why the child does not want to go to school. A child with a TBI may not desire to go to school for reasons related to his injury or perhaps for reasons related to normal peer pressure. Problem-solve the situation by addressing the child's concerns and reassure him that together you will agree on an acceptable solution.

> Some children respond best to cheerleading and hand-holding, while others exhibit more participation when they are quietly reassured and given reasons for each activity.

- Isolation—Some children actually cope by avoiding social interaction and using self-reflection, however, isolation can also be a sign of pathological conditions involving the child's emotional state. Children who have difficulty coping with new limitations or demands placed upon them may shut down and/or withdraw from social engagement. Loss of interest in previous activities and withdrawal may be signs of a developing depressive condition. Encourage social interaction while the child is in the hospital. For example, some rehabilitation units have a policy stating that children must (as medically appropriate) eat meals in the dining room with others. Once the child leaves the hospital, parents and teachers should promote social interaction and facilitate participation in extracurricular activities that are strengths for the child.

- Coping—Some children may seem very mature and appear to be handling everything well, but they may be falling apart inside. They may be martyring their feelings for the good of the family. Remember that sometimes it is the child who seems to have the fewest problems (often a sibling) who falls through the cracks. Parents should spend time with their children individually and on a regular basis to give each child the opportunity to communicate his feelings. Referrals to a psychologist for individual or family therapy may be made as necessary.

Family Adjustment for Children at Different Developmental Stages

Family adjustment and intervention should focus on appropriate activities dependent on the age of the child. Because children of different ages have different needs, the concerns for parents will vary.

The table to the right summarizes the important aspects of a child's life in relation to his stage of development.

Developmental Stages	Important Aspects of Life
preschool	• parent-child interaction • language development
early grade school	• family • socialization with peers • cognitive development
middle school	• independence • academic development • social recreation
high school	• dating • intellectual development • driving • prevocation
young adulthood	• college • vocation • social independence • financial independence

Conclusion

Families have described coping with a child who has a TBI as a "roller-coaster ride." There are bad days and hopefully, many good days. We enjoy working with these children and adolescents within the rehabilitation setting because we can help families deal with the hard times and see the amazing joys that families experience during times of positive recovery.

Improvements that are minor for non-injured children can be monumental for a child with a TBI. We have seen parents cry with joy at the sound of their child's first utterance after an injury, especially when the child says, "Mom." We have also seen parents jump with joy at the sight of their son's first steps following an injury.

One of Dr. Lebby's most memorable experiences in all of the years he has worked in pediatric brain injury rehabilitation involved a child named Julian. When Julian was five years old, he was severely injured in a motor vehicle accident. Julian was in a coma for over two months, and the prognosis for his recovery was poor. Every day, Julian's father took him outside to the playground, sat with him in the sun, and spoke to him as if Julian was awake and aware of the environment. Julian slowly began to show recovery and after five months of hospitalization he was discharged with severe motoric and cognitive impairments. Julian spent the next year in intensive outpatient intervention. Dr. Lebby had not seen Julian since he was discharged from the hospital. One day as Dr. Lebby stepped out of his office, he heard a child shout, "Dr. Lebby...Dr. Lebby...Dr. Lebby." Dr. Lebby turned to see Julian running toward him. Julian jumped into his arms and gave him a big hug.

The memory of Julian, running with his arms open and a big smile on his face while calling out his name, has brought Dr. Lebby pleasure over the many years since the incident. Both Drs. Lebby and Asbell can recall many similar experiences with memorable patients. This is unique to a profession that specializes in assisting patients regain functional independence after a devastating injury.

We hope that you have both enjoyed and learned from our knowledge and experiences involving pediatric traumatic brain injury. Just as we have been able to help others in facilitating positive outcomes, we hope that you too will utilize the information in this book to assist children recovering from complex injuries.

Appendix 11A: Interacting with Children Who Have Disabilities

Able-bodied persons may have difficulty understanding the world of those with disabilities. It is important to be aware of attitudinal barriers when working with children and adolescents who have disabilities.

Language Use (It is important to use "person-first" language.)

- The language you use can result in either positive or negative outcomes. Language use can help change attitudes toward children with disabilities by accurately describing the children, or by reinforcing and perpetuating negative stereotypes and misconceptions.

- A child with a disability is a child first and a child with a disability second. Emphasizing the child, not the condition, demonstrates respect and maintains the dignity of the individual. The child precedes the disability, both figuratively and literally.

Language Use	
Wrong	**Correct**
▪ brain-injured	▪ a person with a brain injury
▪ wheelchair-bound	▪ a person who uses a wheelchair
▪ learning disabled	▪ a person with a learning disability
▪ mentally retarded	▪ a person with mental retardation or a cognitive disorder

Terms to Avoid		
▪ crippled	▪ differently-abled	▪ handicapped
▪ suffers from...	▪ stricken with...	▪ a victim of...

Words like *handicapped, wheelchair-bound,* and *accident victim* may sound neutral or sympathetic, but children with disabilities may find them patronizing and offensive. Someone with a spinal cord injury once stated, "I am not wheelchair-bound. If I tip over, I fall right out of it."

Handicapped has a negative connotation for many people. Handicapped does not refer to the condition of the individual. Instead, it describes barriers (caused by society, the environment, or another person) that negatively impact the functioning of the individual with the disability. Barriers can be:

- physical (stairs, small doorways, hills)
- mental (advanced reading level requirement for written material)
- cultural (language, religion, economics, different life experiences)
- attitudinal (lowered expectations, faulty assumptions)

▌ Things to Consider when Interacting with Someone Who Has a Disability

- **Pity**—Avoid pity. Children with disabilities are not "victims."

- **Reality**—Children should not be described as inspirational or courageous simply because they have a disability.

- **Adjectives, NOT Nouns**—Use an adjective as a description, not a category or group (i.e., *children who are disabled*, not *the disabled*).

- **Terminology**—Terms such as *physically challenged*, *special*, and *differently-abled* are often patronizing. If appropriate, note that a child has a physical, sensory, or mental impairment, and leave it at that.

- **Normality**—Do not refer to children without disabilities as *normal*, because this implies that children with disabilities are *abnormal*. Instead, describe them as children who are *non-disabled*.

- **Germaneness**—Children with disabilities should be treated just like everyone else. You would not mention the physical condition of a person without a disability unless it was germane to the conversation. So, unless the child's disability is relevant, do not mention it.

- **Assumptions**
  - It is better to ask a child with a disability about things you do not know than to make assumptions and be wrong.
  - Do not assume that a child with a disability is incompetent, unintelligent, sick, dependent, or requires help. Most children with disabilities are independent, productive members of society.

- **Normalize Interactions**
  - Do not avoid normal or expected forms of greeting. Most children with limited use of their limbs can still shake hands. If you are not sure, let the child make the first move.

  - The presence of a physical impairment does not necessarily mean a child has a mental impairment as well. Speak directly to the child and leave baby talk for babies.

  - Do not stare, but do not avoid eye contact. Act as you would with a person without a disability.

  - Common expressions, such as *See you later* or *I've got to run*, are not insulting to individuals with disabilities, so do not feel uncomfortable if they creep into your conversation.

- **Offering Assistance**
  - Do not be embarrassed to offer help to a child with a disability, but wait until the child accepts your offer and gives you instructions before you proceed.

  - Do not be offended if a child with a disability does not seek or welcome your help. Most of the time, children with disabilities do not require any help and are fully independent. They may wish to struggle with a door instead of always having it opened for them.

- **Not Everything Is Related to Their Disability**
  - A child with a disability may decide not to talk for reasons that are completely unrelated to his disability. Do not force a conversation if it is clear that the child is not in the mood to talk, and do not assume it is because he has a disability.

  - A child with a disability may seek help in dealing with problems that are the same as those experienced by peers who are non-disabled. If you assume it is related to his disability, you may fail to assist him with the real problem.

Cognitive Disabilities

- Talk in short, simple sentences that are appropriate to the child's cognitive level.

- Maintain eye contact and interact in a manner consistent with that used for those without cognitive disabilities. Avoid childish speech/language, condescending tone, silly remarks, or jokes.

- Ask open-ended questions rather than yes/no or either/or questions. Many children respond *yes* to questions they do not understand, so as not to appear confused.

- When possible, use pictures or diagrams to explain what you mean.

- Do not become frustrated if you have difficulty communicating with the child. Be patient and reassuring.

Language-/Communication-Based Disabilities

- Communication is critical to allow people self-autonomy and independence, and to provide them the means to make their own decisions.

- Just because a child does not have the ability to talk, it does not mean he is unintelligent or does not understand.

- Be patient and make attempts to determine the most appropriate and effective way to communicate with a child. Writing, sign language, pointing to responses that are pictured or written on a board, or even simply blinking for *yes* or *no* are all acceptable means of communication.

- Do not pretend to understand when you don't. Repeat what you think the child said, and if all else fails, use written notes or other means of communication. It is better to spend the time to understand the child than to ignore what he says, as this is disrespectful and communicates that you do not care or that what he said is not important.

- To gain the child's attention, touch him lightly or use some other physical or visual sign.

- If you are using an interpreter, speak to the child you are interviewing rather than to the interpreter. Make eye-contact as you would if you were speaking the child's preferred language.

Visual Impairments

- When meeting a child with a severe visual impairment, identify yourself and introduce anyone else who is present.

- Let the child know when you are leaving and when you return.

- Before trying to shake hands, say something like, "Shall we shake hands?" or reach for the child's extended hand.

- When offering seating, place the child's hand on the back or arm of the chair.

- If walking from one location to another, offer your arm as a guide and alert the child to any obstacles, such as steps, curbs, or low arches.

- If dining, do not feel embarrassed to orientate the child to the location of the silverware or other items.

Use of Canine Companions/Assistants

- The dog is there to work and is trained to attend to the child's needs, not yours.

- Do not treat the dog as if it were the child's pet. Instead, treat the dog as if it is a person—with respect and appropriate distance.

- If you have a relationship with the child and the dog, or if the child informs you that it is all right, you can then interact with the dog.

Physical Disabilities

- Consider a child's wheelchair or adaptive equipment as part of the person. It is not polite to touch or lean on the chair unless the child gives permission.

- When talking to a child in a wheelchair for more than a few minutes, place yourself at the child's eye level.

- Allow children who use wheelchairs or adaptive equipment, such as walkers, to keep the equipment within reach.

Glossary

Active Attention—the ability to hold, process, and manipulate information mentally, while filtering distractions

Activities of Daily Living (ADLs)—refers to basic tasks of everyday life, such as eating, dressing, bathing, toileting, etc.

Akinetic Mutism—refers to a state of consciousness in which the person is alert (has sleep-wake cycles with periods of eye opening), but does not speak (*mute*) and does not move (*akinetic*)

Alexia—the loss of previously acquired ability to read or make sense of written words; often associated with damage to the visual-association areas of the brain in the language dominant hemisphere

Anastomosis—a connection between two structures, vessels, or spaces. The vessels of the brain are interconnected via an anastomosis called the circle of Willis. A pathological anastomosis may occur between an artery and a vein (*arteriovenous malformation* – AVM).

Angular Gyrus—a region of the brain in the parietal lobe that is involved in multiple aspects of language and cognition; located immediately posterior to the supramarginal gyrus, near the superior edge of the temporal lobe

Anterograde Amnesia—a form of memory impairment in which information perceived after an injury to the brain does not become consolidated and stored as long-term memories; a disorder of new learning after a brain injury, even though "old memories" formed prior to the injury remain intact

Aphasia—a disorder of language functioning caused by damage to the brain; can affect functions relating to expressive language, receptive language, or both

Apoptosis—selective cell death as a normal part of brain development; a process which "fine-tunes" the brain to make it work more efficiently

Aprosody—a term that indicates speech is monotone, lacking the emotional quality that is typically communicated by the intonation contours and tonal inflection

Arachnoid Granulations—projections from the arachnoid layer that protrude into the superior sagittal sinus of the brain; allow cerebral spinal fluid to exit the brain and become absorbed into the venous bloodstream

Arachnoid Layer—one of the three layers of the meninges that surround the brain and spinal cord; located between the dura mater and pia mater and separated from the pia mater by the arachnoid space, through which cerebral spinal fluid flows

Arcuate Fasciculus—a neural pathway within the brain that connects language areas in the parietal lobe to language areas in the frontal lobe. Damage to the arcuate fasciculus can cause conduction aphasia.

Astereognosis—inability to identify or recognize objects by touch, often caused by damage to the somatosensory cortex; AKA *tactile agnosia*

Autonomic Nervous System—a part of the peripheral nervous system that controls organs and muscles. There are two branches of the autonomic nervous system: *sympathetic* and *parasympathetic*. Most of the time we are unaware of the regulations of the autonomic nervous system because it functions primarily in a reflexive manner.

Autoregulation—the process in which blood vessels expand and constrict in order to regulate and maintain a constant pressure inside the brain

Axon—the thin projection from a nerve cell that is used to transmit information via electrical impulses toward other cells

Axonal Shear Injury—See Diffuse Axonal Injury.

Ballism—a neuromuscular condition that involves involuntary, abnormal swinging; jerking; or shaking movements of the extremities

Blood-Brain Barrier—blood vessels (*capillaries*) in the brain that have specific epithelium and astrocyte sheaths that act as a barrier to control the flow of substances from the blood supply to the CNS

Brain Herniation—refers to displacement of brain tissue, cerebrospinal fluid, or blood vessels, out of the area that they normally occupy and/or across a barrier or membrane; can involve the brain being pushed through the opening at the base of the skull (*foramen magnum*), which can be fatal if left untreated; swelling can also cause brain tissue to move across dural membranes

Broca's Area—a part of the brain that is involved in speech production; located at the posterior portion of the inferior frontal gyrus and frontal operculum. Damage to Broca's area can result in an inability or deficit involving the expression of speech, often called *Broca's aphasia*.

Broca's-Type Aphasia—an expressive language disorder resulting from damage close to Broca's area; characteristics include reduced speech fluency with many pauses (halting speech), telegraphic utterances, lack of intonation (monotone), impaired repetition, and relatively good comprehension of language; AKA *Broca's aphasia*, *expressive aphasia*, *dysfluent aphasia*, or *motor aphasia*

Central Nervous System (CNS)—the structures of the brain and spinal cord

Central Sulcus—a prominent sulcus of the brain that separates the frontal lobe from the parietal lobe; AKA *Rolandic sulcus*. The primary motor area is located along the gyrus immediately anterior to the central sulcus (*precentral gyrus*). The primary sensory area is immediately posterior to the central sulcus (*postcentral gyrus*).

Cerebellum—involved in the coordination of movement, in the integration of sensory and motor information, and in cognitive processing; located directly behind the brain stem

Cerebral Aqueduct of Sylvius—the canal that connects the third ventricle with the fourth ventricle, through which cerebral spinal fluid flows

Cerebral Spinal Fluid (CSF)—clear fluid that circulates through and around the brain and the spinal cord; acts as a liquid cushion between the brain and the skull; provides buoyancy for the brain; is a reservoir of hormones and nutrients for the CNS

Choroid Plexus—a structure within the ventricular system that produces cerebral spinal fluid

Closed Head Injury—an injury to the brain in which there is no penetration of the skull; often sustained due to blunt or rotational forces to the head

Coma—a sleep-like state in which the person does not speak, follow directions, or show purposeful and functional use of the limbs; with time patients may develop eye opening and even sleep-wake cycles

Concussion—characterized by transient posttraumatic loss of awareness or memory, lasting from seconds to minutes, without causing gross structural lesions in the brain and without leaving serious neurological damage. See Post-Concussion Syndrome.

Confabulation—a condition in which a person with brain damage recalls false information as memories and believes them to be true. Damage to the diencephalon can result in confabulations. Conditions with severe anterograde amnesia and executive dysfunction can also cause confabulations.

Consciousness—a state in which a person has both intact arousal and awareness

Contracture—fixed tightening of muscles, tendons, ligaments, or skin that prevents normal movement and can cause deformity if untreated

Contrecoup—damage to the part of the brain that is opposite the site of the primary blow to the head; contrecoup injuries are caused by movement of the brain inside the skull in the opposite direction of the first impact; can result in more damage to brain tissue at the area opposite the initial contact than the injury sustained at the point of contact (*coup*)

Contusion—a physical injury to the brain which causes hemorrhage of the small blood vessels, resulting in a bruise or hematoma

Cortex—the outermost layer of the cerebrum formed by neurons, cell bodies, and unmyelinated fibers. See Grey Matter.

Cranial Nerves—Twelve cranial nerves, located within the cranium (skull), communicate information to and from the brain, but do not pass through the spinal cord. Some nerves communicate motor information (from the brain), some nerves communicate sensory information (to the brain), and some nerves communicate both motor and sensory information.

Critical Periods—periods in which environmental and/or internal influences have an increased effect on later functioning; referred to as *vulnerable periods* by Dobbing

Coup—damage to the part of the brain that is at the site of the primary blow to the head; injuries at site of impact are called *coup injuries*

Cytotoxic Edema—swelling of the cells of the brain caused by fluid accumulating within the cells; most commonly occurs due to *cerebral ischemia* (cell death due to a lack of oxygenated blood)

Deep Structure—the message the speaker means to communicate, which may be different from the actual words used

Dementia Pugilistica—brain damage caused by repeated head trauma; the cumulative effects of repeated concussions, such as from sports related injuries

Dendrites—tree-like extensions of the neuron cell bodies that receive electrical information from other cells; dendrites form a large network to connect neurons and transmit information to the cell body from axons of other cells

Diencephalon—located deep in the brain (below the cortex); is made up of the thalamus which relays and processes information, and the hypothalamus which controls bodily states

Diffuse Axonal Injury (DAI)—a type of brain injury that causes damage over a widespread area; tearing or shearing forces acting on soft brain tissue results in diffuse axonal injury, which is most evident at the junction between cell bodies and axons, or in transmission pathways; AKA *diffuse shear injury*

Disconnection Syndrome—refers to the interruption of information transmitted from one brain area to another; first discussed by Norman Geschwind (1926-1984)

Dobbing Hypothesis—a hypothesis that suggests brain damage has its greatest influence on development when it takes place during vulnerable periods (i.e., when the cells involved are showing the greatest rate of development)

Dominant Hemisphere—the cerebral hemisphere that is more involved than the other in controlling speech and language skills; in approximately 90 percent of the general population, the left hemisphere is the dominant hemisphere for language

Dopaminergic Pathways—neural pathways that allow for the transmission of dopamine from one area of the brain to another

Dura Mater—the outermost and toughest of the three membranes (*meninges*) that surround the brain and spinal cord

Dysarthria—a speech disorder, characterized by weakness and/or incoordination of the speech muscles. Dysarthric speech is slow, weak, slurred, and poorly articulated.

Dysfluent Aphasia—See Broca's-Type Aphasia.

Dysgraphia—refers to a disorder of writing, characterized by difficulty in expression of language or thoughts via writing; generally refers to an inability to form letters and words via handwriting

Dysnomia—a marked difficulty in retrieving names or words required for oral or written expression

Echolalia—repetition (echoing) of utterances spoken by another person that is typically involuntary and non-communicative

Edema—refers to swelling; generally caused by excessive buildup of fluid in soft tissues of the body and brain

Epidural Hematoma—accumulation of blood between the skull and the dura mater

Episodic Memory—a memory of an event, including the time, place, and emotions associated with the event. Damage to the prefrontal cortex and hippocampus can cause a loss of the ability to store new episodic memories.

Executive Dysfunction—refers to a problem with a person's ability to function in a complex environment; caused by disrupted executive functioning, often as a result of damage to the frontal lobes of the brain

Executive Functioning—the cognitive control and regulation involved in the management of other cognitive processes; allows a person to manage efficiently in complex environments. Executive skills include initiation, planning, organizing, sequencing, abstract reasoning, attention, flexibility of thought, ability to multitask, inhibition, etc.

Expressive Aphasia—See Broca's-Type Aphasia.

Extrapyramidal Motor System—the neural network that includes the basal ganglia and cerebellum; modulates voluntary movements and allows for the production of smooth, coordinated movements

Falx Cerebri—the portion of the dura mater that goes down into the longitudinal fissure, which separates the two cerebral hemispheres

Flat Affect—reduced emotional expressiveness typically characterized by lack of facial expressions, monotone voice, diminished body gestures, and an apathetic general appearance

Fluent Aphasia—a language disorder resulting from damage to Wernicke's area; primary characteristic is an impairment of auditory comprehension; additional characteristics include fluent speech with good articulation and intonation, but with poor semantics, and paraphasic errors; AKA *Wernicke's-type aphasia, receptive aphasia,* or *sensory aphasia*

Focal Injury—damage involving a small, localized area of the brain; often involves bruises (*contusions*), bleeds (*hematomas*), or physical damage caused by penetrating objects

Fourth Ventricle—the diamond-shaped cavity located behind the pons and medulla oblongata and in front of the cerebellum; connects the cerebral aqueduct with the central canal of the spinal cord

Frontal Lobes—cortical areas of the brain that are primarily involved with reasoning, intellect, socially-mediated behavior, modulation of emotions, speech output, and motor functioning

Glia—non-neuronal brain cells that provide structure and nourishment, maintain a constant internal environment by cleaning up debris, form myelin, and participate in signal transmission in the nervous system

Glutamate—a key molecule in cellular metabolism; the most abundant excitatory neurotransmitter in the nervous system; AKA *glutamic acid*

Golgi Type I Neurons—principal neurons which primarily form information pathways from one brain structure to another, or from the brain to parts of the body and back (motor and sensory tracts)

Golgi Type II Neurons—smaller neurons without long axons which function to integrate and process information; found primarily in the parietal (multi-modal or association cortex) and frontal lobes

Grey Matter—areas of the brain composed of the neurons' cell bodies and their dense network of dendrites; includes deeper nuclei of the brain, center of the spinal cord, and the thin outer layer of the cerebral hemispheres known as the *cortex*; lack of myelin covering makes grey matter look darker in contrast to white matter

Gyri—elevated bulges that cover the cortex, giving it a wrinkly appearance

Hematoma—an abnormal collection of clotted or partially clotted blood in an organ or soft-tissue space; caused by a break in the wall of a blood vessel that occurs spontaneously (*stroke*) or from trauma

Hemorrhage—a medical term that means bleeding

Huntington's Disease—a disorder that results in involuntary movements of the body (especially of arms, legs, and face) that significantly affect normal functioning; sometimes referred to as Huntington's Chorea due to dance-like movements some patients exhibit

Hydrocephalus—an abnormal accumulation of cerebrospinal fluid within cavities (*ventricles*) inside the brain

Hypothalamus—a group of nuclei that regulates metabolic activity and controls bodily functions, such as hunger, thirst, temperature regulation, sexual behaviors, and circadian cycles; located just beneath the thalamus

Hypoxia—refers to a lack of oxygen in tissues. *Cerebral hypoxia* refers to a decrease of oxygen flow to the brain, which can occur due to conditions such as drowning, choking, suffocation, cardiac arrest, stroke, head trauma, or poisoning. Brain cells are highly sensitive to oxygen deprivation and can begin to die within four minutes after the oxygen supply has been cut off.

Internal Carotid Arteries—two main arteries that supply blood to the anterior and medial areas of the brain; supply blood to almost all brain areas except the occipital lobes, underside of the temporal lobes, cerebellum, brain stem, and spinal cord

Internal Jugular Veins—transport deoxygenated blood from the brain and head back to the heart

Intraparenchymal (Intracerebral) Hematoma—an accumulation of blood within the tissue of the brain (*parenchyma*)

Ischemia—cell damage or death resulting from a reduction of blood supply to the brain

Ischemic Encephalopathy—cell damage and death caused by a lack of blood flow leading to *hypoxia* (lack of oxygen to the brain)

Kennard Principle—a theory that postulates that brain damage early in development presents fewer deficits than brain damage later in life, due to a high degree of neural plasticity in young children

Lateral Ventricles—the two large, arch-shaped cavities in the cerebrum that produce most of the cerebral spinal fluid

Left Visual Field—an area of vision on the left side of where a person is looking. Information from the left visual field goes to the right side of both retinas and is then sent to the visual cortex in the right hemisphere.

Limbic System—structures (including the hypothalamus, hippocampi, amygdala, fornix, septal nuclei, cingulate gyrus, and mammillary bodies) involved in regulation of emotions and formation/ retrieval of memories; located on both sides of and underneath the thalamus

Literal Paraphasia—production of a word in which a portion of the word contains a phonological error, and at least half of the word is produced correctly; AKA *phonemic paraphasia* or *phonological paraphasia*

Locked-In Syndrome—a neurological disorder involving complete paralysis of voluntary muscles in all parts of the body, except for those that control eye movement

Medulla Oblongata—the lower portion of the brain stem that controls automatic functions and relays nerve signals between the brain and spinal cord

Mesencephalon—also called the midbrain; located below the diencephalon; contains nuclei and pathways that control movement, muscle tone, arousal, sleep, attention, reflexive visual and auditory responses, pain, and species typical behaviors such as mating

Metencephalon—contains the pons on the anterior aspect and the cerebellum on the posterior aspect; pons is an area through which many critical pathways travel, and is also involved with control of sleep patterns and central nervous system arousal; cerebellum is involved with integration of sensory and motor information, muscle tone, coordination, and various aspects of cognition

Minimally-Conscious State—a state of consciousness in which the person generally has intact arousal mechanisms and sometimes appropriate sleep-wake cycles; the person may respond to the environment and exhibit cognitively-mediated behavior consistently enough to allow for a clinician to distinguish it from reflexive behavior

Mixed Transcortical Aphasia—a relatively uncommon type of aphasia caused by damage to the watershed area that surrounds Broca's and Wernicke's areas and the arcuate fasciculus; characterized by severe expressive and receptive language difficulties with intact language repetition

Modified Barium Swallow Study (MBS)—a diagnostic test conducted by a speech-language pathologist and a radiologist to examine oropharyngeal functioning; used to diagnose swallowing problems

Motor Aphasia—See Broca's-Type Aphasia.

Myelencephalon—contains the medulla oblongata, which is involved with many critical life functions, and the spinal cord, which contains communication pathways allowing for information to be transmitted between the brain and body

Myelin—fatty insulation that surrounds neurons and makes up the white matter of the brain; functions to speed up the transmission of impulses along neuronal fibers (*axons*)

Negative Reinforcement—strengthening or increasing the frequency of a particular behavior by consistently stopping or avoiding a negative consequence

Neologism—a word-like utterance expressed by a patient that sounds like a real word, but is not a real word

Neurons—cells that process and transmit neural information; located in the brain, the spinal cord, and the nerves and ganglia of the peripheral nervous system. Neurons have membranes that can be stimulated and allow for the generation and propagation of electrical signals.

Neurotransmitters—chemicals released from a neuron that affect another cell, resulting in the cell becoming more likely to produce an action potential (*depolarization*) or less likely to produce an action potential (*hyperpolarization*). Action potentials allow for transmission of neuronal information.

Non-Accidental Trauma (NAT)—refers to an injury that was intentionally inflicted, such as in shaken baby syndrome, physical child abuse, and battered child syndrome

Occipital Lobes—the primary cortex involved with visual processing; AKA *striate cortex* because it has a striped appearance

Palilalia—a disruption of speech fluency in which there is abnormal repetition of syllables, words, or sometimes phrases/sentences, with increasing rapidity and decreasing clarity and amplitude

Parenchyma—refers to the key elements of an organ, or the substance of the brain. *Brain parenchyma* consists of tissue excluding the meninges and cerebrospinal fluid.

Parietal Lobes—cortical areas of the brain that are primarily involved with the processing and integration of sensory information

Parkinson's Disease—a motor disorder that results from the loss of dopamine-producing brain cells or dopminergic pathways. Symptoms include trembling of the hands, arms, legs, jaw, and face (*tremors*); stiffness of the limbs and trunk (*rigidity*); slowness of movement (*bradykinesia*); and impaired balance and coordination of movement (instability of posture).

Passive Attention—focusing attention on information without the need for active mental manipulation

Pathognomonic—relates to a symptom being characteristic or diagnostic of a particular disease

Penetrating Injury—an injury caused by an object piercing the skull

Peripheral Nervous System (PNS)—the part of the nervous system that consists of the nerves and neurons that reside outside of the central nervous system (CNS); consists of two parts: the *somatic nervous system,* which connects the CNS with the body, and the *autonomic nervous system,* which controls autonomic or automatic bodily functions

Perisylvian Zone—a region around the sylvian fissure that extends from the frontal lobe back to the parietal lobe and down to the temporal lobe. The various language cortices of the dominant hemisphere are located in the perisylvian zone.

Perseveration—involuntary repetition of a behavior or verbal utterance; getting stuck on an mental idea or thought, even when it is no longer appropriate to the task at hand; inability to move from one idea to another when required

Persistent Vegetative State—See Vegetative State.

Petechial Hemorrhages—small amounts of blood that have leaked from capillaries in the brain, often resulting from tearing forces acting on the small blood vessels; often visible as small, round spots on a brain scan.

Phonemic Paraphasia—See Literal Paraphasia.

Phonological Paraphasia—See Literal Paraphasia.

Phrenology—a theory that suggests that one can determine character and personality traits based on the shape of the external surface of the skull

Pia Mater—the thin, innermost layer of the meninges that closely surrounds the entire surface of the brain and goes down into the fissures of the cortex

Plasticity—the ability of the central nervous system to adapt and change in response to environment and/or internal influences

Pons—a structure that is part of the brain stem and the autonomic nervous system; contains many regulatory systems; relays information between the cerebellum and cerebrum

Post-Concussive Syndrome—disruption of the central nervous system that occurs after minor head injury with or without initial loss of consciousness; often caused by diffuse axonal injury and brain contusions. Symptoms resolve after a few days and may include changes in the patient's ability to think and concentrate, headaches, apathy, dizziness or lightheadedness, variable degrees of memory loss, depression, and/or anxiety.

Post-Traumatic Amnesia—the inability to store and retrieve new information

Primary Auditory Cortex—the region of the brain that allows us to process auditory (sound) information; located on the posterior portion of the superior temporal gyrus, temporal operculum, and insular cortex

Primary Motor Cortex—The *precentral gyrus* is the area of motor cortex that controls voluntary movements of the body. The leg area is located at the top and close to the midline. The head and face areas are located at the bottom of the gyrus. The arm and hand areas occupy the largest surface area of precentral gyrus, and are located between the leg and face areas.

Primary Sensory Cortex—receives input from receptors in the body regarding the sense of touch; located in the parietal lobe, just behind the central sulcus

Primary Visual Cortex—the surface of the occipital lobe of the cerebral cortex that receives visual information from the visual pathways

Procedural Memory—refers to the long-term storage of procedures (i.e., how to do things); typically involves motor skills. Procedural memory often remains intact, even with moderate trauma to the brain, resulting in anterograde amnesia for semantic information. Examples of procedural memory include how to swim, ride a bicycle, or play a musical instrument.

Prosody—refers to the melodic intonation of speech and includes vocal stress

Pure Alexia—the loss of the ability to read after a person has acquired literacy; results from damage to the brain or from a lesion that disrupts input from the visual cortex to the angular gyrus. Patients may retain the ability to write and spell.

Pure Word Deafness—a deficit of understanding spoken language; caused by damage to the pathways from the primary auditory cortex to Wernicke's area; causes impaired auditory comprehension of language; ability to speak, read, and write is retained

Pyramidal Motor System—controls voluntary motor movements; consists of upper motor neurons in the primary motor cortex and lower motor neurons in the anterior horn of the spinal cord

Receptive Aphasia—See Fluent Aphasia.

Reticular Nuclei—groups of neurons within the brain stem that control essential functions, such as arousal, sleep, walking, and breathing

Retinal Hemorrhage—bleeding onto the surface of the *retina* (the part of the eye that changes light signals to neural signals); often associated with non-accidental trauma; not as frequently observed in accidental brain trauma

Retinotopic—refers to the organization of the visual pathways in addition to the subcortical and cortical visual areas; organization of pathways and cortices matches that of the retina (e.g., if the image on the retina is a dog standing beside a person, the corresponding activation within the visual pathways and cortex will have a similar organization – cells that respond to the dog will be situated beside cells that respond to the person)

Retrograde Amnesia—a form of memory impairment in which information learned before a brain injury is disrupted; memories that were stored prior to the injury are lost

Right Visual Field—the area of vision on the right side of where a person is looking. Information from the right visual field goes to the left side of both retinas and is then sent to the visual cortex in the left hemisphere.

Secondary Processes—cellular damage that can occur following initial brain damage, such as a blow to the head; usually caused by the release of neurotoxic chemicals following brain injury; can also be caused by swelling, inflammation, and disruption of chemical and electrical processes required for neural functioning

Semantics—refers to the meaning communicated through words

Sensory Aphasia—See Fluent Aphasia.

Shaken Baby Syndrome—See Non-Accidental Trauma.

Shear Injury—See Diffuse Axonal Injury.

Somatic Nervous System—the part of the peripheral nervous system associated with voluntary motor control; consists of peripheral nerve fibers that send sensory information to the central nervous system and motor nerve fibers that transmit information from the central nervous system to the muscles

Source Memory—memory for the context of a previously-stored memory; memory of where and how you obtained information

Spinal Cord—an extension of the brain; consists of similar tissue (neurons and glial); allows for the communication of neural messages to and from the brain and body via the peripheral nerves

Stereotypies—involuntary, repetitive, and sometimes rhythmic or ritualistic movements or utterances

Subdural Hematoma—a collection of blood on the surface of the brain; located between the brain and the dura

Sulci—grooves that cover the cortex, giving it a wrinkly appearance

Supramarginal Gyrus—the part of the parietal cortex at the posterior end of the lateral fissure in the parietal lobe; thought to be involved in word finding and written expression

Surface Structure—refers to the words and punctuation used during verbal communication

Synapse—the gap between neurons, across which neurotransmitters flow to allow for communication from one cell to another

Syntax—a term that refers to the rules that dictate how words or other elements of a sentence are combined so as to be grammatically correct

Telencephalon—makes up the largest portion of the brain; also called the cerebrum; consists of the cerebral cortex, allocortex/limbic system, and basal ganglia

Temporal Lobes—cortical areas of the brain that are primarily involved in memory functioning, emotional regulation, auditory processing, and language comprehension

Tentorium Cerebelli—an extension of the dura mater that separates the bottom portion of the occipital lobes from the top surface of the cerebellum

Thalamus—a large mass of neural cells located on each side of the brain at the top of the brain stem; relays information between the cortex and other parts of the brain and the body

Third Ventricle—a narrow cavity located between the two hemispheres at the level of the diencephalon (i.e., above the brain stem); provides a pathway for the circulation of cerebrospinal fluid

Transcortical Motor Aphasia—a dysfluent aphasia caused by a lesion within the watershed area surrounding Broca's area; Broca's area is not damaged; characteristics are similar to Broca's aphasia, but with good repetition

Transcortical Sensory Aphasia—a fluent aphasia caused by a lesion within the watershed area surrounding Wernicke's area; Wernicke's area is not damaged; characteristics are similar to Wernicke's aphasia, but with good repetition

Unconsciousness—significant alteration of mental status that involves complete or nearly complete lack of responsiveness to stimulation; AKA *loss of consciousness, lack of consciousness*. See Coma.

Vasogenic Edema—swelling due to increased volume of extracellular fluid which comes from blood vessels and accumulates around cells. The fluid can displace the brain and lead to cerebral herniation if it becomes severe.

Vegetative State—a state in which a person has intact arousal and sometimes sleep-wake cycles but deficient awareness (they do not exhibit purposeful behaviors or consistent responses to stimulation)

Venous Sinuses—a network of channels between the layers of dura through which oxygen-depleted blood (*venous blood*) flows, eventually leaving the brain via the internal jugular vein

Ventricles—the four cavities of the brain filled with cerebrospinal fluid. There are two lateral ventricles (one in each cerebral hemisphere), the third ventricle located above the brain stem, and the fourth ventricle located behind the pons and medulla oblongata and in front of the cerebellum.

Verbal Paraphasia—refers to the involuntary substitution of an inappropriate word for an intended word; AKA *semantic paraphasia*

Vertebral Arteries—two main arteries that supply blood to the posterior and inferior areas of the brain; supply blood to the occipital lobes, underside of the temporal lobes, cerebellum, brain stem, and spinal cord

Videofluorographic Swallowing Study (VFSS)—a study in which radiographic images are produced of a patient's swallowing. The patient eats food and drinks liquids mixed with barium, which makes them visible on the video scanner. The images are viewed by a speech-language pathologist and a radiologist to evaluate the patient's ability to swallow.

Watershed Area—the areas of the brain that lie between the middle arteries and the anterior cerebral arteries; prone to ischemic damage, as the tissue has limited blood supply

Wernicke's Area—the part of the brain located in the temporal-parietal region, posterior to the primary auditory cortex; responsible for auditory comprehension

Wernicke's-Type Aphasia—a condition involving disruption of a patient's ability to understand and express language, due to impaired ability to extract the meaning of verbal information. See Fluent Aphasia.

White Matter—the parts of the brain and spinal cord responsible for information transmission; composed of myelinated axons that connect different areas of grey matter to each other and carry nerve impulses between neurons; does not contain dendrites, which are only found in grey matter along with neural cell bodies and shorter axons

X-Ray—a type of electromagnetic radiation that can identify bony structures and detect some disease processes in soft tissues; primarily used for diagnostic radiography (i.e., to identify potentially treatable conditions). Computed axial tomography (CT or CAT) uses x-ray technology to produce images of the brain.

Anderson, V., Northam, E., Hendy, J., & Wrennall, J. (2001). *Developmental neuropsychology: A clinical approach.* Philadelphia: Taylor & Francis, Inc.

Brodmann, K. (1909). *Vergleichende lokalisationslehre der grosshirnrinde in ihren principien, dargestellt auf grund des zellenbaues.* Leipzig: J.A. Barth Verlag.

David, R.B. (2005). *Child and adolescent neurology.* (*2nd Edition*). Malden, MA: Blackwell Publishing.

Hagen, C., Malkmus, D., Durham, P. (1972). *Rancho Los Amigos Levels of Cognitive Functioning.* Downey, CA: Rancho Los Amigos Hospital.

Lezak, M.D., Howieson, D.B., & Loring, D.W. (2004). *Neuropsychological assessment. (4th Edition).* New York: Oxford University Press.

Love, R.J., & Webb, W.G. (2001). *Neurology for the speech-language pathologist. (4th Edition).* Boston: Butterworth-Heinemann.

Rizzo, M., & Eslinger, P.J. (2004). *Principles and practice of behavioral neurology and neuropsychology.* Philadelphia: W.B. Saunders Company.

Shonkoff, J.P., & Phillips, D.A. (2000). *From neurons to neighborhoods: The science of early childhood development.* Washington DC: National Academy Press.

Spreen, O., Risser, A.H., & Edgell, D. (1995). *Developmental neuropsychology.* New York: Oxford University Press.

Teasdale, G., & Jennett, B. (1974). Assessment of coma and impaired consciousness: A practical scale. *The Lancet*, (ii), 81-83.

Whishaw, I.Q., & Kolb, B. (2003). *Fundamentals of human neuropsychology. (5th Edition).* New York: Bedford, Freeman & Worth Publishing Group.

Recommended Resources

http://www.asha.org/public/speech/disorders/Traumatic Brain-Injury.htm
American Speech-Language-Hearing Association (ASHA)
ASHA is the professional, scientific, and credentialing association for more than 123,000 members and affiliates in the United States and internationally. ASHA is dedicated to promoting the interests of and providing services for speech-language pathologists; audiologists; and speech, language, and hearing scientists, and advocating for people with communication disabilities.

http://www.biausa.org
Brain Injury Association of America (BIAA)
Founded in 1980, BIAA is a national organization that provides information, education, and support to assist the 5.3 million Americans currently living with traumatic brain injury, their families, and the professionals who work with them. The BIAA also has a network of more than 40 chartered state affiliates, as well as hundreds of local chapters and support groups across the country.

http://www.cdc.gov/ncipc/tbi/TBI.htm
Centers for Disease Control and Prevention (CDC): National Center for Injury Prevention and Control.
The CDC, a federal agency under the Department of Health and Human Resources, provides health information for your general knowledge. TBI definitions, epidemiological information, etiology, and symptoms are outlined on the website.

http://www.carf.org/
Commission on Accreditation of Rehabilitation Facilities (CARF)
CARF, an independent, nonprofit organization founded in 1966, reviews and grants accreditation services nationally and internationally on request of a facility or program. The organization's focus is on ensuring that services meet patient and family needs for quality and the best possible outcomes. CARF has rigorous standards, so the services that meet them are among the best available.

http://www.ndrn.org/
National Disability Rights Network (NDRN)
NDRN is a nonprofit membership organization for the federally-mandated Protection and Advocacy (P&A) Systems and Client Assistance Programs (CAP) for individuals with disabilities. Together, the P&A/CAP network is the largest provider of legally-based advocacy services to individuals with disabilities in the United States.

http://www.nichcy.org/pubs/factshe/fs18txt.htm
National Dissemination Center for Children with Disabilities (NICHCY)
NICHCY serves the United States, Puerto Rico, and the U.S. Territories. It provides families, students, educators, and others with information on topics regarding children and youth with disabilities (birth through 22 years). NICHCY also provides information regarding IDEA (the law authorizing special education), No Child Left Behind (as it relates to children with disabilities), and research-based information on effective educational practices.

http://www.ed.gov/about/offices/list/osers/nidrr/index.html
National Institute on Disability and Rehabilitation Research (NIDRR)
NIDRR is one of three components of the Office of Special Education and Rehabilitative Services (OSERS), a branch of the U.S. Department of Education. NIDRR conducts research and coordinates programs in an effort to promote full inclusion, social integration, employment, and independent living of individuals of all ages with disabilities.

http://www.neuro.pmr.vcu.edu/
National Resource Center for Traumatic Brain Injury (NRC for TBI)
The NRC for TBI provides relevant, practical information for professionals, persons with brain injury, and family members. Additionally, they publish books, manuals, and kits for children and adults that address issues related to TBI.

23-07-987654321